Talking with Patients

MIT Press Series on the Humanistic and Social Dimensions of Medicine

Stanley Joel Reiser, General Editor

Talking with Patients

Volume 1:
The Theory of Doctor-Patient Communication

Eric J. Cassell

The MIT Press
Cambridge, Massachusetts
London, England

This book was set in Baskerville by Asco Trade Typesetting Ltd., Hong Kong, and printed and bound by The Murray Printing Company in the United States of America

Library of Congress Cataloging in Publication Data

Cassell, Eric J., 1928–
  Talking with patients.

  (MIT Press series on the humanistic and social dimensions of medicine; 1–2)
  Includes bibliographies and indexes.
  Contents: v. 1. The theory of doctor-patient communication—v. 2. Clinical technique.
  1. Physician and patient.   2. Interpersonal communication.   3. Medical history taking.   4. Medicine, Clinical.   I. Title.   II. Series.   [DNLM:
1. Communication.   2. Physician-Patient Relations.   W1 MI938M v. 1–2/
W 62 C344t]
R727.3.C38   1985   610.69′6   84-26120

Volume 1
ISBN 0-262-03111-6 (h)
       0-262-53055-4 (p)
Volume 2
ISBN 0-262-03112-4 (h)
       0-262-53056-2 (p)

To my beloved and loving children,
Justine and Stephen

Contents

Foreword

Medical encounters begin with dialogue. Language transforms the experience of illness into subjective portraits painted by the patient. The patient's account of events leading up to the sickness, of sensations felt indicating something is wrong, of interpretations giving the symptoms meaning are all part of the patient's story. The patient's role as narrator in the drama of illness has declined in the twentieth century. This is due to the growing dominance of technologically centered techniques of medical evaluation in which the views of the patient become largely irrelevant, if not obtrusive. The numerical results generated by the analytic technology of the modern medical laboratory, the graphic depictions of illness produced by machines that monitor the electrical actions of the body, the neatly ordered printouts of clinical data developed within modern computers—all these data seem free of the bias and subjective opinion of a person and possess the objective characteristics of evidence we call scientific. Where, then, is there room for the patient's story, told from an admittedly biased viewpoint and delivered to the doctor with all of the inaccuracies, inconsistencies, and omissions characteristic of human memory and speech?

In this two-volume treatise Eric Cassell has set out to fill a large gap in the literature of medicine by giving a systematic account of how language works and how such an understanding can be applied to transforming communications between patient and physician into precise tools of evaluation and therapy. There are few more important tasks for contemporary medicine than this one. In medicine's vigorous pursuit of the biologic knowledge of disease, patient's and their lives have been left out, partly because the method of learning about them—human communication—has seemed an art incapable of describing and thus teaching about with the exactness possible when examining a biochemical event.

Combining information provided by over a thousand hours of tape-recorded conversations between physicians and patients, extensive research into the theories of linguistics, and the experiences of a long career as a clinician, Eric Cassell has formulated a conceptual view of medical communication and a format for its practical clinical application in patient care. He has given form to this subject, and provides a clear agenda of study to enhance our communication skills now and to learn more about them through future research.

It is crucial for modern medicine to establish a balance between understanding general biologic processes that make us ill and understanding the illness as experienced and produced by the patient. To learn of the latter, the verbal and nonverbal elements of human communication in medical care must be understood and mastered. These volumes lead us toward this goal in a more comprehensive way than any other work in the modern literature.

Stanley Joel Reiser

Acknowledgments

The story of this book started in 1973 with a grant request to the Robert Wood Johnson Foundation. I was interested in studying the belief structure of medicine—the system of beliefs and values concerning illness, the body, doctoring, and the doctor-patient relationship on which medical practice is based. Margaret Mahoney, then vice-president of the Robert Wood Johnson Foundation, provided a planning grant.

Bernard Sussman and then Ellie Schoenbaum (recent college graduates then, and now physicians) were research assistants as we prepared a proposal that might allow an approach to so complex a problem. Two things seemed plausible. First, the beliefs and values held by patients and physicians should make themselves known in their spoken interaction; therefore it would be necessary to record and study doctor-patient conversation. Second, I would have to learn about values and the way in which people think about values. A mammoth research proposal ensued for studying how medical students acquire the belief and value structure of medicine, and how they learn to think of values during their training. Miss Mahoney and Terrance Keenan (also of the Robert Wood Johnson Foundation) patiently helped me pare the ideas down to manageable size. They believed correctly that concentrating on dialogues between patients and their physicians would be both possible and productive.

With their funding I set out to find how these conversations should be studied. It was disconcerting to discover how many different camps there are in the field of linguistics. All over the country, however, linguists of many different pursuasions generously gave me their time and interest. I found that there had been few studies of doctor-patient conversation; indeed, the study of natural conversation was still in its early stages. George Miller, at the Rockefeller University, suggested that I speak to Bruce Frasier at Boston University. Dr. Frasier, understanding that my primary concern was not the study of linguistic phenomena but their application to medical education and practice, helped plan an effective approach. He remained a consultant to the project for its duration, and there are few his equal at quickly identifying and clarifying linguistic issues. I am in his debt for all his help and for suggesting Lucienne Skopek as linguist-in-residence. Dr. Skopek gave me an education in applied linguistics. Although the first chapter, on paralanguage, is most directly the result of her written collaboration, her ideas and thinking can be found throughout this book. Research of this type is never solely cerebral; she reviewed many hundreds of hours of tape recordings in order to discover the phenomena reported in this book and to find the best examples. In addition for three years she kept our academic laboratory in running order, for which I am most grateful.

Robert Mayer was the research assistant most identified with the solution to the innumerable technical problems associated with taping, cataloging, storing, and retrieving more than a thousand hours of doctor-patient conversations. In addition his creativity and hard work added much to the quality of tape examples employed for teaching.

The initial research was successfully completed, and the Robert Wood Johnson Foundation provided further support for the development of a curriculum to teach the theory and skills of medical communication to students and physicians. Margaret Mahoney and Terrance Keenan were again very helpful. In the development of curricular materials, Constance Wilkinson Gianniotis provided assistances too numerous to count, including editorial, creative, and technical help. In this later phase of the work, Elliot Susseles, Betsy Guenthner, and Lachlan Forrow (both the latter now physicians) also provided assistance. Nancy McKenzie, a philosopher, joined the laboratory under a one-year grant from the Blum Foundation. Her clearheaded and incisive thinking and questioning proved of inestimable help in resolving some of the conceptual problems that had to be surmounted. Dr. Skopek was also an invaluable aid in bringing the literature of linguistics to bear on our work.

In writing this volume, I have provided a bibliography of books that I believe will introduce the reader to the study of the spoken language. Linguists and philosophers of language will quickly note gaps, but the bibliography is not intended for them. Others who wish to study the subject in greater depth will be able to go on from these sources.

In carrying out this project, the focus was always on developing concepts and skills that could be taught and that would be effective in clinical medicine. Therefore I am especially in debt to the many students who have taken these courses over the last several years. Their enthusiasm and involvement has provided both motivation to move forward and specific criticisms on which to base improvements. Over eight hundred patients were kind enough to sign consent forms and wear the microphones that made possible the unique collection of doctor-patient recordings on which this book is based. I am in debt to the many physicians (especially Peter Dineen, Stanley Birnbaum, Gerald Klingon, and Morton Colemon) who, knowing that their previously private conversations with patients would be subject to scrutiny, offered themselves and encouraged their patients to participate. From October 1974 to December 1975 the tape recorders were in my office documenting every interaction between me and consenting patients. (I stopped when I began to believe something was "real" only if it had been recorded.) I must thank my office staff, Esther Hyman, Maria Lopez, and Nancy Levy, for so gracefully putting up with the inconvenience. As always I am in debt to my patients for their willingness to participate and for tolerating this and the other things that have allowed their care to be the ultimate test of the ideas in this book.

The National Library of Medicine (Grant LM00056-01) povided the funds that made writing this volume possible. For the tedious and hard work involved in typing transcripts of lectures, I wish to thank Nancy Levy. Corinne Standish accomplished the exacting task of transcribing the examples as they appear in the text. Dawn McGuire, supported in part by the Commonwealth Fund, has been my research and editorial assistant during the completion of the book. Her many skills and keen thought are everywhere evident. I am especially grateful for the encouragement of Dr. Stanley Reiser which helped bring the book to completion. Walsh McDermott, so helpful throughout my career, understood what I was after and how important it might be to clinical medicine. His support and encouragement was always of tremendous importance, and his death in October 1981 was a great personal loss.

During the past three summers, when the bulk of this book was written, my wife and I have spent August in a small country cabin with two computers and their paraphernalia as our word processors. My wife has always been my surest guide and critic; for this volume she has also been an editor. What would I have done without her? Even as I write this, she is deep in her own work on the other side of the room. There are surely better vacations, but never a better partner.

Talking with Patients

Introduction to Volume 1

This book is based on four premises about clinical medicine: doctors treat patients, not diseases; the body has the last word; all medical care flows through the relationship between physician and patient; and the spoken language is the most important tool in medicine. Because not every physician would agree with these beliefs (although most would accept the primacy of the body), a little history is necessary to situate this book and the ideas in it.

During the 1930s my grandmother saw a specialist about a melanoma on her face. During the course of the visit when she asked him a question, he slapped her face, saying, "I ask the questions here. I'll do the talking!" Can you imagine such an event occurring today? Melanomas may not have changed much in the last fifty years, but the profession of medicine has. I believe medicine is in the midst of fundamental and exciting changes; it is evolving toward a profession in which the primary concern of physicians is with sick (or well) persons rather than merely their diseases. Indeed, this is probably the most profound shift in medicine since the concept of disease, as we know it, came into being in the 1830s.

Medicine has always been a profession of action: doctors do things to their patients. When the primary focus of medicine is on diseases, the important acts of physicians are, generally speaking, acts of discovery. In his book *Doctor and Patient*, Dr. Lain-Entralgo tells the story of the brilliant clinician Skoda making rounds. Skoda held forth at the bedside of a patient, displaying his usual diagnostic skill. At the end one of his assistants asked what should be done for the patient. Skoda impatiently brushed the question aside as irrelevant! Because of the lack of effective therapies in his day, one might understand Skoda's posture. However, only a few years ago the same attitude was expressed by a resident who told his students that only three things were important in medicine: "The diagnosis, the diagnosis, and the diagnosis." In view of the importance of diagnosis and research, it is no wonder that the heroes of the disease era were heroes of discovery—primarily research scientists.

In the last few decades, with the advent of modern therapeutic effectiveness, we have changed from a profession of discovery to one in which intervention is primary; now the acts of physicians are acts of intervention. It should be no surprise that the heroes of an interventionist medicine are often surgeons, and the status of research scientists has faded (a state of affairs that could compromise progress in medicine). While one would think that the behavioral guidelines and the basic concepts and skills that doctors acquire during their training would be truly different in an era of intervention, compared with those aquired in the era of discovery, this does not yet seem to be the case. In emphasis and curricula, with a few notable exceptions (particularly among the new medical schools), medical education today is monotonously similar to my own education thirty years ago. Lack of change in the educational agenda is one of the reasons that our exciting and successful interventionist technology continues to have many problems in its application.

Although physicians can often do marvelous things for a liver or a cardiopulmonary system, what is good for the liver, the heart, or the lungs is not always good for the patient! Symptomatic of our difficulties is a patient with end-stage ventilatory failure, whom all know is as good as dead, still hanging from a respirator which no one has the nerve to turn off. Everybody is uncomfortable about such a situation: students talk about not wishing to play God; the hospital administrator fears a law suit; the house staff wonders how many more times they will be called on to resuscitate the patient; the attending physician avoids talking frankly to the patient or the family; and the family guiltily wonders how much longer all this will go on. When I was a student, my professor of surgery described an exploratory laparotomy on a patient with bowel obstruction in the days before long tubes. He said, "As I watched them trying to stuff all that distended bowel back in the belly, while it kept popping back out, I thought, 'This just can't be the way things are meant to be.'" Thinking about patients like the one just cited I feel the same way. Difficulty in judging how best to use the new knowledge causes trouble for patients and their families and creates emotional and professional strains for physicians as well. Not only does conventional training fail to prepare physicians to mediate these strains, the orientation of training is itself responsible, at least in part, for the undiscriminating use of medical technology. The attitude taken by some physicians is, "If it *can* be done, it *should* be done."

Classical science taught that to understand the whole, whether it be a human or a laboratory mouse, one should break it down into observable parts, isolating (in a controlled fashion) the aspect to be studied. The results of such research, when they are put back together, are believed to give an understanding of the whole organism. The science that underlies the brilliant accomplishments of modern medicine, and that all physicians are taught, is based on such reductionist beliefs. It is obvious to most, however, that despite past achievements the complexity of human existence with its creativity, desires, hopes, aspirations, as well as oppression, war, poverty, and misery has not yielded to the methods of science. Rather than either pretending that reductionism is working when it is not, or eschewing science for some mystical approach, concerned scientists have searched for alternate scientific methods. A whole new way of thinking about the complex wholes that physicians deal with—persons, families, and communities—a theory of "general systems," has come into being. The emphasis in this book derives from systems thinking: physicians dealing with sick patients must always try to find out how the pathophysiology that bears on the illness is expressing itself at the whole human level, as well as at the organ and cellular levels.

During this period, when doctors are beginning to confront the dilemmas of technical versus humane medicine, the general public has also changed its attitude toward medicine and its practitioners. Increasingly dissatisfied with reductionistic principles, people are seeking what is popularly referred to as "holistic" medicine. Although most people are not sure what holism is, they are quite clear about what it rejects: the treatment of patients by physicians as though they were merely objects, diseases, or malfunctioning body parts. As practiced now, however, holism frequently seems to embrace chiropracty, "megavitamin therapy," and other alternative therapies that do not seem to many of us either holistic or even particularly useful. These deficiencies should not keep one from recognizing the unmet needs and the social force for change represented by holism.

If the sick person is to be the focus of medicine, then new concepts, skills, and guidelines for behavior are needed. In medicine we do not simply describe the procedure for an appendectomy and then leave students to their own devices. We define appendicitis, base the definition on anatomy and pathology, demonstrate how it manifests itself, how the diagnosis is made, and how to treat it. Similarly it is not sufficient to tell a student or physician to treat sick persons and not just their diseases. Without the necessary definitions, tools, and skills all that has been created is a moral injunction, like the story of the Good Samaritan—"Go and do thou likewise." When a person fails to fulfill a moral injunction, that person generally ends up taking the blame and feeling badly. Then, despite good intentions, patients are not better off, and doctors feel like failures. This is frequently what happens today when physicians start their internships. They are supposed to care about their patients as "persons," use their "feelings," and be "open" and communicative. Given the fact that they have no specific training in this aspect of patient care, however, that they are overwhelmed by work, and that they are usually rewarded for technological rather than interpersonal skills, the young physicians' sense of inadequacy may defeat their good intentions.

From time immemorial there have been physicians who were extraordinarily adept at working with patients—taking histories, establishing rapport, achieving compliance with even the most unpleasant regimens, being sensitive to unspoken needs, providing empathetic support, communicating effectively, and even getting paid after the illness. This expertise, usually called "the art of medicine," is acquired by most through years of experience. Some doctors, nevertheless, are more skilled with patients than others; because of this it is frequently said that the art of medicine is a matter of "intuition" and is unteachable: "You either have it or you don't."

I am convinced that the art of medicine can be studied and taught in a systematic and disciplined manner. Critics often act as though the words "systematic and disciplined" are applicable only to science and are incompatible with "art." Ludwig van Beethoven, judging from his notebooks, was extremely systematic and disciplined, as were Michelangelo, Pablo Picasso, and probably every other fine artist. With regard to teaching an art, although talent and intuition may be essential, even child prodigies have teachers and work constantly to refine their skills. In the absence of disciplined effort prodigies would surely not realize their promise.

The art of medicine is composed of abilities in four different but interrelated areas. The first is the ability to acquire and integrate both subjective and objective information to make decisions in the best interests of the patient. The second is the ability to utilize the relationship between doctor and patient for therapeutic ends. The third is knowing how sick persons (and doctors) behave. Finally, the central skill on which all the others depend is effective communication, the subject of this book.

This book is about the spoken language in medicine, about conversation between patients and doctors. The chapters that follow go into considerable detail about how the spoken language actually *works* in medicine—how it does its job. We would never dream of teaching physical diagnosis to students lacking a background in anatomy and pathology. It is important to know not only what hepatomegaly due to metastatic cancer feels like but *why* it feels the way it does. Similarly it is a great help, when listening to heart sounds, to be able to visualize the heart in action. Although physicians in training will have a chance to feel the nodular liver of malignancy and to hear the murmur of mitral stenosis, the next liver and the next murmur will not present themselves in the same way or in the same setting. One must not only have experienced fingers and ears but the knowledge to interpret sensory information when it varies from that encountered on previous occasions.

Because the way a person speaks is an intimate and integral part of that person, the spoken language differs from other tools and skills in medicine. Digitalis glycosides work the same way whether the doctor prescribing them is shy or bold, sensitive or overbearing; the drug's action is separate from the doctor. If a doctor is teaching the use of a sigmoidoscope and says, "Never push the 'scope forward unless you see a hole," it does not matter what kind of a person you are for the strategem to work. Suppose, however, that the interviewing instructor tells you, "Walk straight in and say, 'My name is Doctor Osler and I'd like you to tell me the story of your illness.'" Perhaps you can do that, but if you are uncomfortable, the words may sound wooden and artificial. For you it may be necessary, for example, that the patient give some sign of approval before you can feel at ease asking questions. "Hi, Mrs. Friendly, may I sit down? Thank you. My name is Bill Osler. Could you tell me the story of your illness, please?" Speech is part of the presentation of self, and a speaking style that is foreign to you will not work. When, however, you understand the function of the utterance—what you want it to do—then the phrases can be successfully adapted to your personal style.

One would think that the spoken language would have been subject to intense scrutiny, given its importance. Yet the scientific study of natural conversation is a relatively new discipline. The basic difficulty with such study derives from the fact that language is fundamentally and irreconcilably different from other objects of scientific inquiry. Science has been successful because of the ability of scientists to study in controlled isolation, simple, linear, cause-and-effect parts of more complex wholes. This produces "dyadic" statements of the type with which we are all familiar: "If A, then B."

Starling's law of the heart is of that type, as is the All or None rule of nerve conduction. Explanatory principles are easily constructed when phenomena can be characterized in terms of dyads, or sets of dyads.

Language, however, is totally different; it is irreducibly triadic. Words do not merely stand for things, as in "Apple is a word that stands for the firm, fleshy, edible fruit of the tree, *Pyrus malus*." How about "She's the apple of my eye," or "One bad apple spoils the whole barrel," or even "Adam's apple." If words merely represented things in the same manner that a thermometer reading represents a certain temperature, then the study of language would proceed in a nice orderly manner. But whereas the thermometer functions independently of persons who might take an interest in its reading, words do not; they represent not only something "out there" but the person using them as well. With exceptions that will be discussed in the text, words always stand for something *to someone*. The irreducible triangle consists of a word, the thing it stands for, and the person for whom it has that meaning. Complications arise because there are almost always variations between the meanings of the same words for different people. Since one cannot verify in objective terms what is going on inside the mind of another, the problem of personal meaning has thus far proved impenetrable.

Fortunately all the features that make the spoken language opaque to science provide opportunities for clinicians. Human illness is, in fact, triadic in the same manner as language. Diseases, when isolated and confined to their afflicted cells, organs, or enzyme systems, may be quite constant in the manner in which they express themselves, and we have instruments that measure their activity, just as a thermometer measures the kinetic behavior of molecules. However, each *illness* caused by a given disease is unique and differs from every other illness episode because of the *person* in whom it occurs. Even when a disease recurs in the same individual, the illness is changed by the fact that it *is* a recurrence; it now carries the associations and the history of the previous episode. Though it is obvious that genetic makeup or changes in immune response can alter the reaction to disease, as can diet, personal habits, and level of physical conditioning, the presentation, course, and outcome of a disease can also be affected by whether the patient likes or fears physicians, "believes" in medication or abuses drugs, is brave or cowardly, "self-destructive" or vain, has unconscious conflicts into which the illness does or does not fit, and so on. These features are part of the illness, for illness is not only a physical event but a "meaning event" as well. Throughout the book the reader will see examples of patients attaching meaning to symptoms and illnesses. Indeed, there is no event that befalls humans to which meaning is not attached. It is the triadic nature of human illness that makes the art of medicine so vital; if every patient were the same, then merely to know the disease would be to know the illness.

The material in this book is drawn from hundreds of hours of natural conversations between doctors and patients in offices, hospital rooms, clinics, and emergency rooms. These hours were distilled in turn from well over one thousand hours of recordings involving many physicians and more than eight hundred consenting patients taped in 1974 and 1975. (In contrast to most previous studies of doctor-patient communication, only a small minority of these recordings involved clinic patients or doctors in training.) My staff and I attempted to apply the existing knowledge in linguistics to the specific problem of doctor-patient communication. However, every idea and concept had to meet two simple tests: was it relevant to conversation as it actually occurrred, day to day? and was it relevant to better patient care? (Tape recorders are like cameras; they merely record what is, whether flattering or not. Listening to a conversation in which you have tried a new way of talking can indicate success or failure in short order. I strongly recommend that you tape your own conversations with patients. Nothing will enlarge understanding more rapidly—this has been my own experience and that of my students.)

The object of the analysis of these recorded conversations was an increased understanding of medicine, not of linguistics per se. Nonphysicians and students of language who may read this should be aware that, although much of what is presented here clearly has wider theoretical implications for the study of the spoken language or applicability to other fields such as law or education, this is a book about medicine, by a physician, for physicians and students of medicine. (Similarly I have ignored some of the issues that have exercised linguists interested in doctor-patient communication because I do not believe that they have utility in the care of patients.)

The examples, besides illustrating issues in communication, also involve actual cases and approaches to the care of patients. The reader will become closely acquainted with how I practice medicine, what I believe the nature of the relationship between patient and physician should and should not be, and even how I treat certain illnesses. In addition the personal approaches of other physicians are exemplified.

When I first started listening to recordings of other physicians in their offices, I was pleased to hear that the same things, some of them quite strange, happened in their offices as in my own. Doctors who have listened to me with my patients have expressed the same sentiment. The practice of medicine is a very private matter. The most intimate aspects of a patient's life are revealed in physicians' offices, ranging from what kind of underwear is worn (or not) to what the person secretly thinks about other family members, as well as the overtly sexual matters that are usually associated with the word "intimate." At times the doctor is as much exposed as the patient; for this reason I admire the doctors who put aside their reservations to wear my microphone. Consequently readers should understand that they are privy to information shared by few in the past. For the same reason and because it has a single author, this book will be unavoidably idiosyncratic. Despite the drawbacks of this personal quality I hope the reader will find learning about how another doctor works as interesting as I do. Because this approach is neither quantified nor treated statistically, it may cause discomfort to physicians who have been raised on numerical data and taught to avoid the anecdotal. I believe that there is *no* other equally effective or realistic manner, however, to approach the study and teaching of communication between doctor and patient in the clinical setting. Indeed, the recitation of cases—telling stories—has been a way to teach medicine that has survived through the ages because nothing else does the job as well. In fact recently scholars have begun to direct attention to the stories about patients used in teaching because they convey a kind of information that can be transmitted in no other way. Because the information presented here is personal, subjective, or anecdotal does not mean that it cannot be studied in a systematic manner that will allow generalization beyond the particular instance. Examining the music of a particular composer, for example, will reveal aspects that are unique to the composer's style. Studying the same music, one can demonstrate the rules of form and composition that apply to music generally. So it is in this book: examples drawn from the interaction between two people reveals things about these two people as individuals and also about interactions and communication in general.

It takes time to become adept at using the spoken language as an effective medical tool; readers should be patient with themselves, but persistent. It may require many months before you begin to hear people shift to impersonal pronouns when they describe their illnesses or unpleasant events, as described in chapter 2. But once you become aware, you will hear the phenomenon everywhere. The secret of mastering the spoken language in medicine is simple—just keep at it.

Remember, you cannot avoid using the language; the question is whether you will use it to its best advantage. Let me recommend again that you tape your own conversations with patients. Modern tape recorders are so small and unobtrusive that it is generally a simple thing to do. Remember to ask the patient's permission. Patients generally do not mind as long as they know that their privacy will be maintained. (The appendix describes the techniques for recording in greater detail.)

When I was a medical student I bought a copy of Bailey's *Physical Signs in Clinical Surgery*. It was full of wonderful pearls of wisdom about physical diagnosis. It sat by my bedside for years, and I would often pick it up and read wherever it happened to open. On many occasions what I learned from Bailey has worked for me. I began to buy copies and give them away as gifts for my students, so that they too should come to love the lore of clinical medicine. (You'd do better to buy the earliest editions you can find; the later editions are weaker.) It is my hope that students and physicians will find that the more medicine they know, the more this book has to offer, and that it too will be worth revisiting.

References

Bailey, H. *Demonstrations of Physical Signs in Clinical Surgery*. Ed. by A. Clain. 16th ed. Bristol: Wright, 1980.

Lain-Entralgo, P. *Doctor and Patient*. Trans. by F. Partridge. New York: McGraw-Hill, 1969

Laszlo, E., ed. *The Relevance of General Systems Theory*. New York: Braziller, 1972.

Percy, W. *The Message in the Bottle*. New York: Farrar, Straus and Giroux, 1975.

1

Paralanguage:
The Music of Language

In this chapter, the first on how we know what people mean when they speak, I am going to discuss paralanguage. Paralanguage (or paralinguistics) is the music of language: those nonword phenomena, such as pause, pitch, speech rate, and intonation, that tell us so much of what someone wants to say.

In this chapter I am also going to begin to teach you to listen to the spoken language in a new way. Before going further, however, let me address the difficulties that arise in writing about a process that can only be heard. I have attempted to overcome these problems by illustrating my points with examples from natural conversation transcribed so that you can translate, to some extent, what you read into what you might hear. In later chapters I believe you will find it quite feasible to learn the skilled use of the spoken language by reading about it. In this chapter, however, I am like an instructor trying to describe music for a class without an instrument to play it on. And I cannot even use my hands to talk to you. Therefore, wherever it is really necessary to hear the examples, I suggest that you try reading them aloud.

Crucial to skilled listening is the ability to separate the observation (what was said, and how) from the interpretation (what does the speaker mean). Before I go into more detail, let us look at some examples.

Our first example is a woman who had been operated on some months before and was found to have a carcinoma of the colon metastatic to the ovary. She is admitted on this occasion because of back pain and ascites. She is a short, plump white woman of sixty-seven, with an attractive smile and a certain sparkle. At this moment she is telling me, in response to my questions, about the history of her illness. She has a Boston accent, a leisurely speech rate, and a strong straightforward intonation, with a somewhat nasal drawl, as though some southern accent has crept in. The vocal pitch is in the low range for a woman:

Dr. Dineen said—while he was going to be very honest with me— that, there was a possibility of a—colostomy—
Mm-hm

—which I of course dreaded very much. But, it would be a temporary one, just for two weeks.
Mm-hm.

And, uh—anyway, it didn't turn out that I needed a colostomy and the— the, uh, tumor ate a hole I guess, in part of the colon and was working itself AWAY from the colon.
Mm-hm.

So Dr. Dineen was called in because the ovaries had been affected. One, but he- he, he removed both.
Mm-hm.

And, uh, Dr. Dineen removed the— ah, tumor—
Mm-hm.

and, uh, then we had to wait for the tests—
Mm-hm.

—and, uh—of course it WAS malignant.
Mm-hm.

But, uh,—they got everything and all the radiologists and everybody said that there was no— no uh, concern for treatment and everything was fine.

She said that last sentence in a pleased and definite manner, the way you might say, "It was a nice party and everybody had a good time."

But, see what she says just *one* day later. The only thing that has occurred is that she has had a number of diagnostic studies: X rays and a sonogram.

Gone is the firm deliberate full-sounding speech of yesterday. Instead, her voice is thin and wavery and high-pitched. The speech rate is slower, and the syllables are drawn out. We call that whining:

I get about an hour relief today . . .
From what, huh?
The Darvon . . .
All right, we'll giv—that's not strong

But she ... she gave it more often—
Did you, uh- Have you ever taken Percodan?
Yeah, 'n it's TERrible.
What does that do to you?
It makes me very high and it doesn't take the pain away—
All right. Have you ever taken—
Years ago it did.
Mm-hm. Have you taken Talwin? Have you ever taken—
Aw-ful, y-es.
What does that do to you?
It-makes-me-so-nervous and—
And what does Demerol do to you?
—no appetite.
What does Demerol do to you.
I—don't—remember ... 'bout Demerol—
All right I'm going to give you some Demerol and some Thorazine together, side by side, so you don't get nauseated from it and so you get some—
I—hope—I—don't—go out of this world with the—
With what?
I'm afraid of d— the Demerol.
What from? Why are you afraid of that?
Well—does it have a reaction like Talwin?
Make you nervous?
The Talwin, ooooohhh— I was in— an— with every—thing— the—pain—was—still—there—
All right, now—
Mm-hmmm (whines and moans)
You know what you're doing now? You're sittin' there bein' dragged around by your back.
Ahmmm—

The differences between her speech on day 1 and day 2 are primarily in her paralanguage. The intonation, pitch, pausing, speech rate, and intensity have all changed. Most listeners on day 2 would find her disagreeable to listen to, whiny and annoying. Without knowing why, they would begin making interpretations and forming opinions (mostly negative) about her. And chances are, because of her effect on them, they would not adequately control her pain. If physicians know that it is her tone of voice that turns them against her and makes them discount her complaints, they can act on this knowledge, just as knowing that only certain gram-negative organisms produce that odor does not make an abcess smell better, but it increases the chance that a physician will act correctly.

The patient's tone of voice is an example of paralanguage. Let us now examine the concept of paralanguage and discuss its importance in understanding language use in medicine.

What Is Paralanguage?

In its broadest sense paralanguage can be defined as all nonverbal symbolic communication activity, including gestures and facial expressions. In this discussion, however, paralanguage will be considered in a narrower sense, as nonword features of spoken language: (1) pitch, (2) stress, (3) intonation, (4) pause, (5) speech rate, (6) volume, (7) accent, and (8) voice quality.

Let us define these terms.

1. *Pitch.* Pitch is directly related to the speed of vibration of the vocal cords. The faster the vibration the higher the pitch. Its absolute range refers to the level of pitch characteristic of a particular class of speakers (male, female, child) or to the pitch a speaker may use in special circumstances. Variation in pitch is mainly a feature of a spoken phrase. Conventional pitch modulations for English speakers help mark the function of an utterance. They may indicate

a question (rising pitch): You are going?
a statement (falling pitch): You are going.
a nonfinal phrase (level pitch): You are going ...

2. *Stress.* When words are spoken, they are given a stress by changing pitch or making a syllable louder or longer. In some words more than one syllable is stressed.

When words are combined in a phrase, only one of the syllables in the phrase receives the primary stress, and the other stresses are reduced. That is, the syllable that has received the main stress when the word is isolated may have only secondary stress in a phrase. Any unexpected change in stress, any shift of stress from a normally stressed element to one not normally stressed, creates a constrastive or emphatic stress:

usual stress: She is going home.
contrastive stress: She is going *home.*

A speaker may emphasize words or phrases that are important by shifting or increasing their stress. Consider the previous example:

"Have you ever taken Percodan?"
"Yes ...'s TERrible."

Or, later

"It makes me SO nervous ..."
(Instead of the more usual, "It makes me so NERVous.")

Travelers asking directions in a foreign language are frequently frustrated not by lack of vocabulary but by errors in stressing the syllables of a name. On one occasion I could not make a French policeman understand that I wanted to get to rue NaPOLeon. Finally he realized that rue NapoleON was my destination, and he quickly directed me. My annoyance was tempered by wondering how long it would take me to understand where a foreigner in New York wanted to go who asked for MaDIson Avenue, instead of MADison Avenue.

3. *Intonation.* Synchronized pitch and stress variations within a sequence of syllables (phrase, clause, sentence) create intonation patterns.

4. *Pauses.* Speech interruptions occur in a speech segment and consist of silence or nonspeech sounds.

5. *Speech rate.* In the simplest sense speech rate concerns the number of syllables per unit time. However, speech rate must also take account of pauses, and a more accurate definition is: the ratio of the number of syllables produced to the number and length of pauses.

When the ratio of syllables to pause length is varied ever so slightly, most of us know immediately that there is something different about that speech. One of the tasks involved in learning to use language in medicine is to move this skill from intuition to awareness.

6. *Volume.* Conventionally one associates volume with the loudness of someone's voice. However, I might also have used the term *intensity*, because this feature of paralanguage is not loudness alone (the number of decibels) but includes the sense of force behind the words. Volume (or intensity) plays an important role in the perception of intonation.

7. *Voice quality.* An important clue to a speaker's identity is the quality of his or her voice (hoarse, clear, nasal), but this characteristic is likely to be influenced by affective states and emotional conditions. A

change in voice quality often makes us aware that someone has become ill.

8. *Accent.* We use accent here in reference to the different pronunciation of sounds and the paralanguage characteristic of speakers with different dialect and language backgrounds.

Paralanguage accounts for the acoustic shape of human speech; it is the unusual use of paralanguage that causes us to recognize computer-produced speech as nonhuman: mechanical, hollow, incomplete. Paralanguage is particularly powerful since it can change entirely the literal meaning of words. For example, whether the phrase "Boy that was a great dinner" will be interpreted as a compliment or an insult will depend to a great extent on the paralanguage of the speaker. Particularly in everyday conversation, paralanguage eloquently communicates nuances of mood, emotions, and intent. Because paralanguage is the feature of speech least likely to be under the speaker's complete conscious control, attention to paralanguage will often reveal information not obtainable from words alone.

It is crucial to realize that paralanguage is intrinsic to the comprehensibility of the spoken language. Each language uses paralinguistic features differently. In English, for example, variations in pitch change the meaning of a phrase; in a "tone" language like Chinese, on the other hand, variations in pitch change the meaning of a word. Speakers of the same language (or dialect) share agreements about the meaning of paralanguage and learn to interpret what they hear according to social, cultural, and individual norms. Language would be useless were this not the case.

For our purposes the significance of paralanguage comes from the contrast between expected and unexpected usages. Any deviance from the expected norm—a pause that sounds too long, an unusually fast speech rate, a flat intonation pattern—affects a listener in a particular way. A listener may "like" or "dislike" the way someone sounds. The listener may find the speaker "stupid" or "educated," "nervous" or "depressed," "reliable" or "unreliable"; the listener may identify the speaker as a New Yorker, a southerner, a foreigner. These impressions are largely formed below awareness, on the basis of a person's use of paralanguage. Physicians must become aware of the fact that we pass such judgments on our patients. We must learn to recognize what we actually hear before we can competently address our patients' problems.

Observation and Interpretation

The distinction between the observation and the interpretation of spoken language, that is, the distinction between what we actually hear and what we interpret it to mean, cannot be overemphasized. This difference is often difficult to recognize, because the two processes occur almost simultaneously in the communication process and are usually blurred. Generally, when we listen to speech, we interpret it immediately (that is, attach meaning to it). If at a later time our interpretation is challenged, we may not remember the actual data, the words and the sounds of the speech, that led to our interpretation; consequently we are unable to correct our error or defend our interpretation. This blurring is especially true of paralinguistic features.

From very early childhood we learn to interpret nonverbal cues. Indeed, mothers generally speak words and sentences whose literal meanings cannot be known to their young children—even infants—but employ strikingly exaggerated paralanguage in an attempt to get their meanings cross. It is common for adults speaking to young children, even those old enough to understand words, to switch into the same exaggerated paralanguage: "Oh whaat a preetty dress, aren't youuu a biiig girrll!"

Through this early experience children come to know the conventions of their language: what a long pause means, what a rise or fall in pitch means, and so on. They learn to attend carefully to these cues and to interpret their meaning. Very rapidly children learn to recognize sadness, anger, happiness, not so much from the words speakers use but from the way they say the words. By the time speakers are fluent in their native language, they do not discriminate between what they actually hear and what they believe to be the meaning.

It is an error to equate an observation with an interpretation because the hearer takes the meaning of the sounds to be what those sounds mean to the hearer, not necessarily what they mean to the speaker. This may be good enough for ordinary conversation—in fact it is, or there could be no ordinary conversation—but it is not sufficient for a physician who is trying to use what the patient says as a basis for action. A slight margin of error in the meaning of speech is no more tolerable than a margin of error in the meaning of heart sounds.

Using heart sounds as an example also emphasizes the fallacy of substituting interpretation for observation. In teaching physical diagnosis, we try to stress the importance of describing what the murmur sounds like—its location, place in the cardiac cycle, pitch, duration, quality. The terms *murmur of aortic insufficiency*, *mitral murmur*, *ejection murmur* are not a substitute for such description. Someone hearing or reading these phrases does not know what the murmur sounded like. They know what the doctor thought; but what if the doctor was wrong? In like manner it is not sufficient to write that "the knee demonstrated acute arthritis." We want to know whether it was red, hot, tender, or swollen. And if so, how much of each. Arthritis is an interpretation. We want the original data, so that later findings from the same patient, or other patients, can be compared. In the same way we expect trained listeners to remember language data (what the spoken words were and how they sounded) separate from any interpretation of meaning. With paralanguage, it means hearing fast speech, long pauses, high pitch, rising pitch, before interpreting these as "nervous," "depressive," "sad," or "ironic." This separation is fundamental for skillful use of language in medicine.

Listening to and Interpreting Paralanguage

Let us return to the woman in the first example. Because of the changes in her paralanguage one could say she was a whining, frightened-sounding patient. Whining is a language behavior most people find unpleasant, not to say irritating, and it is a style to which listeners react strongly. Because of this reaction listeners are prone to ignore what is actually said. Instead, interpretations about the speaker's behavior are commonly made. Simple ones like "She's acting like a baby," to more psychological interpretations, "She's just trying to make us dislike her." The net effect of these interpretations is to minimize the perception of the patient's distress. Suppose in fact she is "just trying to make us dislike her"; does that tell us how to act toward her, or what to give her for pain? We behave in this manner because such paralanguage usually accompanies other behavior whose overall message is "Nobody can help me." This makes physicians feel powerless, which tends to drive them away from patients. My interpretation of the feeling of powerlessness is also a psychological interpretation and is, on the face of it, no better than any other. The difference is that the first set of interpretations—"She's acting like a baby"—rarely come from a thoughtful response to sensory data, which was fully heard and appreciated. Instead, they are spontaneous and usually untrained responses to the expression of negative emotion in a patient. Rarely do such responses lead to effective action.

The second set of intepretations—"Patients who behave like that generally feel powerless"—consists of conscious responses to observed behavior, which are not only related to the actual clinical situation but, more important, can lead to effective action. Further these latter interpretations are based on remembered consciously processed information. We can disagree about our interpretation of the facts but not about the facts themselves.

Any obstacle to the observational process should be identified and removed—whether this be merely a personal bias, the fact that the listener finds some listening experiences unpleasant, or a belief that a certain psychological formulation so well fits the facts that further listening is deemed superfluous. Inattentiveness also leads inevitably to flawed observation, and it matters little whether attempts to justify this are simplistic or sophisticated. In ordinary conversation it is quite normal for other events, or even passing thoughts, to distract one's attention; in a professional setting, however, that is not acceptable. Fortunately attentive listening, as difficult as it is, becomes much easier with experience and effort and eventually becomes a part of everyday ongoing behavior.

I cannot stress too strongly the fact that attentive listening is a skill born of practice. As the months go by, you will find that increasingly you hear *only* the speaker and that your mind has become free of distracting thought.

How "Subjective" Is What the Listener Hears?

The question of the "subjectivity" of the spoken language always comes up, and this seems a good place to discuss the issue.

The simplest answer is that, yes, all spoken language is subjective. But to which meaning of that complicated word "subjective" do we refer? There are at least three meanings that concern us, and these are frequently confused in medicine.

The first meaning is represented by: you see "red" and I see "red," how do I know that you see what I see? The answer is that I do not know whether you see or hear what I see or hear. We are both able to *use* the information of our eyes and ears in the same manner, however, and with training, we can both be taught to discriminate and agree on very subtle differences in shades of red.

The second meaning of "subjective" more commonly referred to in medical practice is: you say you have a "bad" pain in your back, and I do not know what "bad" means.

There is a third meaning of the word "subjective" which requires comment. The meaning of things to me is part of my subjectivity. We both read the room thermometer as 68 degrees Fahrenheit, which is an objective measurement. Yet I think it is too chilly, and you think it is just fine. These personal meanings are subjective. We both see a cat; a cat is a cat, but it means nice, cuddly animal to you, and to me it means wheezing and allergy. The cat is an object; the meanings are subjective. We will deal with this latter aspect of subjectivity in chapter 4.

The spoken language, it turns out, is subjective in every one of these three senses of subjectivity.

Pauses

At this point I would like to examine a paralinguistic feature in greater detail. I have chosen pause because it is one of the simplest aspects of paralanguage to learn to hear. Not only can pause be unequivocally identified, it also serves to bring the listener's attention to other features of paralanguage.

"Silent pauses" have been distinguished from "filled pauses." Silent pauses are actual silences occurring between words, phrases, and sentences. Filled pauses are sounds such as "uh," "um," "er," that fill hesitations in speech.

Goldman Eisler (1968) suggests that pausing occurs when speakers make cognitive choices, that is, when speakers decide what they will say next. Pausing is shorter when the thought to be expressed is simple and longer when the thought is complex or original. Most of Eisler's work, however, has been carried out in a laboratory setting and may not reflect what goes on in natural conversation. As well as being correlated with cognitive processing, pauses may serve other functions. For instance, filled pauses may occur when speakers wish to "hold their place" in a conversation. Their "uh's," and "um's" indicate that they want to "keep the floor" and do not want to be interrupted (Maclay and Osgood 1959). Investigators have shown that pause is correlated with emotional states, such as anxiety and depression (Mahl et al. 1956, 1959, 1964, 1971; Pope et al. 1970).

Learning to Interpret Pause Length in Conversation
Even if we cannot always reach agreement about the meaning of pauses, we can perceive them as they occur and thus reach agreement in terms of our common observation of a common event. For example, we would have little difficulty in agreeing that the following is a long pause—not a short or a medium length pause. (Recite it with the pause length. Then try other pause lengths.)

If you're very tired, is the pain worse?
... (five second pause) ... No.

Recite the same segment with shorter or longer pauses and listen to
the effect of varying pause length on your perception of the answer.
You will quickly note that any pause over two seconds seems long.
This judgment is, however, affected by how slowly or rapidly the
question is asked. Thus the perception of pause length is related not
only to the time occupied by the pause but to the speech rate of the
questioner. Change the answer to, "No, it only seems that way." Now
recite the question and answer at different rates, also varying the
pause length, and you will be aware of how much information can go
into the judgment of pause length.

Now I shall present several examples of natural conversation,
so that you may begin to develop a sense of pauses between words
and utterances. Initially, focusing particularly on pauses may make
it relatively more difficult to concentrate on the accompanying
words—this device is suggested to train you to become more conscious of the occurrence of pauses on the one hand, and of their
meaning, on the other. I found, when I was learning to listen, that I
had to tell myself to listen to the pauses (or the speech rate, pitch, etc.)
and when I did, the words receded into the background. Focusing on
the words, I would not be conscious of the paralanguage. The experience is similar to concentrating on the techniques of camera work
at the movies and thus losing track of what is actually going on.

In the following examples the pauses are mainly used for people to
make cognitive choices. The speakers are responding to standard
questions in the course of a medical history, and their pause lengths
will vary depending on the complexity of the questions.

Where were you born?
I'm laughing hysterically. (Laughter) New York City.

Where were you born?
Ah, New York City.

You were born in Scotland?
Mm-hm.

Where were you born, Helen?
Uh, in New J— you mean here?
Mm-hm.
In this country, New Jersey.

While we do not know what is occurring within the speaker during pauses in speech, we can observe that questions eliciting simple information are, as a rule, quickly answered. When this general rule is violated, as in the last example, we know it to be odd ("Uh, in New Je—, you mean here? In this country? New Jersey?"). A trained listener might infer that something else is going on in the patient's mind that might require further questioning.

The form of the questions used to elicit information can, in themselves, increase or reduce pausing. "Where were you born?" is a simple question asked and routinely answered in life, one that should be answered with little or no hesitation. On the other hand, the question, "you weren't born in New York, were you?" contains not only a request for simple biographical information, but an inference on the part of the speaker, which the hearer will have to take into consideration before replying.

Note the following questions and answers.

Are your parents alive?
Well my mother's alive, my father's deceased.
How old was your father when he died?
Fifty-five.
What did he die from?
A stroke.
And your mother is how old?
Ah ... sixty, I guess.
Is she in good health?
Yes. She had-ah, heart palpitations. She suffered when my grandmother died.

It is interesting to realize that, in this example (and generally), the speaker responds more rapidly when giving information on the dead parent's age than that of the living. Perhaps this is because the deceased parent's age is fixed and requires no further computation or perhaps for more intricate reasons. We do not know why, it is merely interesting. But the fact is there, whether we know why or not.

Please note the following questions and answers:

How much do you drink?
Liquor?
Yeah.
Very little.

How much do you drink—alcohol.
Very little—maybe a beer at night.

How much do you drink alcohol?
Oh...socially. Maybe tw...well, on the average I'd say maybe three nights a week? Two drinks a night? You know, cocktails—

How much do you drink alcohol?
Um...virtually nothing unless it's like two in the morning and I can't fall asleep, but I mean, if we're out to dinner I might have tomato juice or maybe sherry, I-I...
Mm-hm.
Only at night if I'm reall— if I have insomnia which— is very frequent, you know (laugh) I'm tense.

And how much do you drink?
Well, uh, I've cut it down but I did drink a bit, but I never drunk anything else but su-Scotch and water and, eh, now I have knocked off altogether now.
When you were drinking, would you drink a fifth a day?
Oh no!
Half a—
Fifth a day?
Yeah.
I guess I could drink a pint a day—
Mm-hm.
...well, that's a— let's see...you mean a fifth?
Yeah, I mean a whole bottle.
Oh, no, no, (laugh) no. No, that would do me about two days, three days.
Hm.

How much do you drink alcohol?
... I'd say, four to six ounces a day.

Do you drink any, uh, how much do you drink alcohol?
Oh, I haven't had a drink since Friday. I had two or three drinks Friday.
Usually.
I usually have one, two beers in the evening. The weekends, maybe two or three drinks.

How much do you drink—alcohol?
Welllll, ... I may have one drink of an evening—'n possibly two. Maximum. Unless—
Mm-hm.
—it's a very very special occasion 'n it'd be three. When I say "an evening," I mean a Saturday night! But during the—
Right.
—week there is no drinking at all.

In these examples, pause length is variable. The question asked requires more than simple recall of stored information: time is also needed to formulate the wording of the response. In addition the patient's answers also involve the presentation of self. The answers tell the questioner not only about alcohol usage but also about the kind of person the patient is. This is because information about some personal behaviors, such as alcohol use or sex, are inherently value laden: hearing the answer, the listener may form an opinion about the patient. Respondents know this, and it influences not only the content of their answers but also their paralanguage, particularly their pauses. In a later chapter I will show how the problems raised by value-laden questions can be overcome.

Next note an example of filled pausing occurring while the speaker is actively selecting a train of thought:

There are two problems that I'm going to cope with tonight.
Yeah.
One is your heart, and one is fear.
.... Yeah.......... I know uh, ... I know I'm probab— I

may be one of the world's worst reporters, of my— uh—symptoms you know.

Mm-hm

And, uh . . . . but . . . I'm trying to sort of organize them sitting over here, you know.

Mm-hm.

I know it was pretty regular until about last—you have the date over here when you made a—a date for me to come in and take an exercise tolerance test.

In the following example the speaker has chosen the thought to reply appropriately to the given questions but then pauses to select particular words:

What kind of pain was the residual pain?
Uh, gee, I— I can't even, uh, ... w— it was in the same spot, I just felt—
Mm-hm. Dull, achey, burning?
Dull. Sort of dull pain.

As physicians, we constantly hear people searching for particular words to describe pain. You may ask, "What kind of pain was it?" and they say, "A pain." "But what *kind* of pain?" We need to know specifically what kind of pain because the difference is crucially important. Physicians have different words to describe pain for the same reason that Eskimos have a great number of words to describe snow—courses of action depend on being able to distinguish between snow type 14 and snow type 7, or between an exquisite pain, and a dull, achy pain.

Patients, having no such need to acquire a large, precise body sensation vocabulary, take more time choosing words to describe themselves or their experience, or else select words that are simply less precise. This may be one of the reasons that physicians routinely offer a list of descriptive words to patients, asking them to choose among them. In the first segment, the doctor asked, "What kind of pain was the residual pain?" and when the patient proved unable to give a quick response, the doctor supplied the word choice—"Dull? achy?" The choice of words requires time.

In addition to the pausing that provides time for language formation, choice of thoughts, or choice of words, speakers sometimes pause in order to censor what they say. A classic example of censoring occurs in the following utterance where it takes the speaker only a fraction of a second to substitute a more acceptable version for an expletive. While we may not know exactly what phrase "Like the . . . . . dickens!" replaces, some very swift censoring does seem to be going on.

You look good, actually, you know?
Well, thank you. I've been working like the . . . . . dickens, shall I say.

Pauses in conversation have other functions as well. Pausing is used for effect, for emphasis, for timing. Often, the pattern of pausing is characteristic of someone's speech. Comedians and actors are masters of controlled pausing, using it as a device in humor or drama. Pausing is sufficiently predictable so that variations from expected pause provide the attentive listener with important clues about the behavior of speakers.

Interpreting Pause in Doctor-Patient Conversations

Earlier I mentioned studies that showed pause to be related to cognitive processes occurring at points of uncertainty in speech. Silent pauses, in particular, seem related to a search for words that most accurately convey the speaker's meaning. As in "What kind of an illness was your hepatitis?" (pause) ... "Very inconvenient!" Hesistant speech, with frequent silent or filled pauses, often accompanies the creation of new or complex thoughts. Usually unambiguous words such as yes or no are preceded by short pauses. Fluent speech (where pauses are short and infrequent) accompanies the presentation of familiar phrases or ideas that have been in the front of the speaker's mind for some time.

You can play a simple game to make these points. In a group of people, ask someone the make (or make and year) of his or her first automobile. There is almost always a pause before the response. Then ask someone else the same question. The second person will usually answer without pause, as though the question asked of the first person caused the second to pull the information from memory so that it is "up front." Conversely, of course, a speaker answering readily with information that should require memory-searching time, betrays that the information has been previously brought from memory. "Has anyone in your family had cancer?" (no pause) "My father's sister, her two sons, my mother's aunt and uncle, and my grandmother's great-uncle." Hearing this, we have reason to believe that cancer has been on that patient's mind.

Armed with these concepts, you can begin to hear and interpret pauses (or their absence) which occur unexpectedly in doctor-patient communication.

Note this next question and the pause, which precedes the respondent's verbal reply:

Do you test your own urine?
...Uh.......

According to the concepts just discussed, we already possess several items of useful information. The question asked requires a seemingly simple yes or no answer. Since the expression of simple thoughts requires the least amount of cognitive processing time, a pause in this situation is unusual. The speaker is having some kind of difficulty providing information that should be simple to process. In the complete interchange, the patient spontaneously reveals the information (that he has not been testing). The trained listener, however, should have been alerted to this possibility on noting the unusually long pause.

Do you test your own urine?
... Uh....... I have the facilities for doin' it but I haven't been doing it.
Have you done it at all in the last few months?
.......No.

Note this next question, pause, and answer, and see if you can make a judgment about the reliability of the information given.

Do you test your own urine?
Yeah.

This information sounds reliable; it is, however, a transcription that presents a successful lie. (We know this on the basis of information revealed later in this particular interview.) It is a successful lie because the verbal and nonverbal content of the message fulfills listeners' usual expectations for a simple answer to a matter-of-fact question. (The patient answers "yes" without hesitation). Were the speaker to pause (as in the previous question), to alter pitch remarkably, or to reply "rhubarb" instead of "yes" or "no," we might be alerted to question further.

Now this conversation continues:

Do you test your urine?
Yeah.
And you're not running sugar? How often do you test?
...... Twice a day.... Test paper.

As in the first example we note that an odd pause precedes a seemingly simple answer. This pause seems out of place because it expresses uncertainty on a topic about which only seconds before certainty was expressed.

In both cases the point of paying careful attention to pauses is to enable the trained listener to note unexpected pausing when it occurs and to take this as a cue to question further, either immediately or later in the interview.

The next example is a reworked version of a doctor-patient conversation. When I began tape-recording physicians, I made it clear that I would not use actual examples of doctors and patients to illustrate poor listening or poor language use. I did this for two reasons. First, although most patients were not bothered by the microphone, physicians usually expressed discomfort. They were sure I was trying to "catch" them in poor communication; they were, in a word, self-conscious. Second, I do not think important things are best taught by using negative examples. We do not demonstrate surgeons nicking the aorta in order to emphasize the need to be careful. Nevertheless, listening to some negative examples can be a useful experience. In order to include these true examples, and at the same time keep faith with the physicians recorded, for the example tapes I created a fictitious medical practice—of the Doctors John and Mary Dolt who were rerecorded for teaching purposes employing actors. The following example was recorded at the Dolt Clinic:

Hi there, Mrs. Bevis. How are you doing?
Just fine.
You know, I saw your husband here last week.
Oh?
Yeah. Jeez, from the look of his penis you two must have really been going at it!
..... oh .... Yah—

It is the long pause in Mrs. Bevis' response (along with lowered volume and raised pitch) that undercuts the literal meaning of her reply. We know that these manifestations carry unusual meaning because, when we listen to her speak, we hear that they are not part of her normal speech production; instead, they appear suddenly in response to the physician's last question. (In addition, of course, the doctor is committing an unforgiveable breach of confidence.)

Please note the next example and decide whether the information elicited is reliable. Base your interpretation on specific features of the speech and on your own experience as a speaker and a listener:

How are you doin' with the booze?
.... Same.
Keeping it down?
Mm-hm.
Good.

Many of those who listen to this tape-recorded example believe this patient is untruthful, that he is drinking more. The listeners are wrong; the patient is truthful. In fact from the paralanguage alone (or even the words themselves), no clue is offered. Here, the listeners are probably forming their judgment not on the paralanguage (or the specific words) but on the oft-stated belief that drinking histories and smoking histories are not trustworthy. The patient said he is not drinking much so automatically that he is considered to be lying. If you, as a physician, believe this, you should not bother to ask in the first place. If, on the other hand, you are aware that drinking histories must be obtained with care, just because they are sometimes un-reliable, you will frame your questions with care and observe the answer carefully prior to your interpretation. If necessary, repeated questions can be used to clarify any doubts. The best form of such questions is discussed in chapter 6. I will note here, however, that it is wise to avoid any question that will elicit yes or no answers of questionable reliability. After all, once a patient has said "no," if you do not believe the person, it is hard to keep questioning without calling that patient a liar. People do not like to be treated like a liar, even (or especially) when they have just lied.

There is a further point. Limited inferences can be drawn from a single piece of evidence. Precisely because the ways people use lan-guage *are* variable, *are* flexible, any generalization must be applied with flexibility. To assert rigidly that "every time a patient pauses before giving information to a physician, he is attempting to lie or conceal," or that "an unusually rapid response means concern," would not only be presumptuous but also inaccurate. This is another reason I stress separating observation from interpretation, separating the facts as experienced from the judgments made about these facts. The phenomenon we are observing in this case is the pause itself; any judgments we make on the basis of this evidence, any conclusions, must be drawn with a light touch and must be supported by additional information.

The practical reasons for maintaining this light touch should be clear from the examples already offered. In one case the patient was telling the truth, and in the other the patient's use of pauses concealed the truth. For a listener to have formed a rigid judgment of either patient's character, or credibility, on the basis of these pauses alone would be foolish; each piece of information revealed in language is just that, and no more: one piece of information. Making premature attempts to decode and to construct patterns to fit bits of information is a misleading pastime. I believe it is more accurate and more useful to pay intense attention to verbal and paralanguage phenomena as they occur—to try to observe simply and precisely, suspending your instinct to make judgments in anticipation of facts. Further, when on the basis of perceived information you make a judgment, it should be done with the understanding that a contradictory piece of information may come to light at any time.

Physicians as Speakers

All the rules that apply to patients as speakers apply to physicians when we talk. Remember that in learning to listen, you are learning what, in a sense, you already know. You already know that frequent filled pausing can mean uncertainty. What you are learning is how to use this information *consciously*. Your patients also know these things, although usually below awareness. Consequently the attentive listener also listens to himself or herself.

Patients pay very close attention to what their physicians say to them, including their paralinguistic cues. Note the filled and silent pauses in this example, where a doctor is speaking to a woman just back from the recovery room following a thoracotomy for an unknown mass in the chest. At the operation she was found to have an inoperable carcinoma of the lung.

Well, you got a tumor there that's gonna be, ah, treated with radiation. And it's not gonna need to be—removed. It's gonna stay right where it—
Another tumor?
Huh? Not "another tumor." What does "another tumor" mean?
I thought he cut it out.
No, ... uh, in its position it gets treated with radiation.
. . . Benign?
Hm? No. Its not. But, um, . . . it's a—, um, gonna get a—, ah, a good response to radiation. Um, uh—you're gonna get a— a good response, your're, uh, you're gonna be a—, uh, well again. Um, you're gonna get a good response.

Because of the physician's repeated use of pauses, the message that comes across is that the doctor is not telling the truth. The words being used are words of certainty; the hesitant paralinguistics communicate uncertainty. The filled pauses undercut the verbal meaning of the message.

Although the physician is trying to reassure the patient, the unskilled use of the spoken language produces precisely the opposite result. Because of the physician's hesitance, suggested by the physician's pausing, the meaning that comes across is that the patient is *not* going to be well again and that the patient is *not* going to get a good response to radiation.

In the clinic, and on the floors, as doctors talk to their patients, you will hear mistakes like this all the time—physicians whose language transmits contradictory meanings. If you ask, "Did you tell the patient what was wrong?" the doctor will answer, "Sure." If you ask, "Did the patient believe you?" he may also answer, "Sure," quite unaware that the patient has been left with a very clear impression that the doctor just lied. Patients are extremely polite; they will not tell you that you have just lied, or that they do not believe what you said. But if you sound like the physician in this example, that is the judgment they will make. Fortunately, the last example is an altered one. Here is the original:

Well, you got a tumor there that's gonna be, uh, treated with radiation. It's not going to need to be removed. It's not gonna need to be removed. It's gonna stay right where—
Another tumor?
Huh? Not "another tumor." What does "another tumor" mean?
I thought he cut it out?
No, uh, in its position it gets treated with radiation.
. . . Benign?

Hm? No. It's not. But it's gonna get a good response to radiation. You're gonna get a good response. You're going to be well again, you're going to get a good response.

The speech of this physician sounds straightforward, and indeed, the *only* difference between the two examples is in the speaker's use of pauses. We physicians need to be aware of paralinguistic elements *as we speak*: if we wish to convey a certain meaning to a patient, we must use not only the appropriate words but the appropriate paralanguage.

This example may raise the question of whether it is also an example of a successful lie. In point of fact this patient *will* do as well with radiation as with surgery. With either treatment her chances of long survival are very poor. Her thoracotomy was in the spring of 1975. She was then radiated. In August 1975 a solitary cerebral metastasis was removed. Until a month or two before her death, in June 1980, the patient was alive, well and functioning—married and maintaining her previous employment.

Even if the answer given was an outright lie, however, this course of action might be chosen for a particular patient. Having carefully assessed the situation, you may decide that a lie is the best policy. The important thing, then, is that if you are going to lie, it had better be convincing. In this particular case the patient did get a good response and was well for five years. What "well" means may vary from person to person; in this person's case "well" meant returning to a functioning life. In general, that is the object of medical care—to return persons to function.

Vocal Paralinguistic Features

I have discussed pause extensively, but paralinguistic features such as pitch, stress, speech rate, and intonation patterns are also major ways of communicating information.

Psycholinguistic studies consistently have indicated that vocal cues affect a listener's perception of the speaker's personality, emotions, and affective states. Several studies suggest that listeners have stereotyped conceptions about the relationship between a speaker's personality and his or her use of paralanguage (Allport and Cantril 1934; Fay and Middleton 1940; Hunt and Lin 1967) and, more specifically, have found that speech rate correlates closely with listeners' judgments of speakers' personality characteristics (Brown et al. 1972, 1973, 1975). Others have shown that speakers can convey various affective meanings by varying their speech rate, pitch, and intonation, even under experimental conditions when the messages being sent were devoid of verbal content (Davitz and Davitz 1959; Davitz 1964). The expression of "controlled" anger, for instance, is usually accompanied by slow speech rate, low pitch, and frequent pausing (Eldred and Price 1958; Pope et al. 1970). Using the spectrograph to analyse speech has confirmed that the most consistent acoustic manifestations of anger, fear, and sorrow are perceived in terms of pitch variations. In angry outbursts, pitch is higher than in neutral situations; in sorrow, pitch is very low (Williams and Stevens 1974). These findings have been utilized in the popular development of so called vocal "stress analyzers," meant to detect when the speaker is lying.

We also know that there are paralinguistic variations along cultural and socially defined norms. For instance, dialect variations may be accompanied by speech rate, volume, and/or pitch which differ from our expected norms. A Southerner's speech is usually slower than a New Yorker's. Nonnative speakers of English may superimpose the paralinguistic features of their mother tongue on English, resulting in unusual paralinguistic patterns. Socially defined norms are also significant, especially when paralanguage and word content are contradictory, as in irony and joking. Furthermore individual differences exist, even among speakers of the same cultural and linguistic background. Some speakers speak fast, others slow; some voices are pitched higher than others.

Most listeners recognize the meaning of these differences but are not aware of the original data that led to their interpretation. What is important is to hear the features that make you perceive a speaker one way or another and to recognize the differences you may encounter when listening to a particular speaker. In other words, you should be able to say, "This woman's pitch level rose," or "His speech is much faster than usual." These changes in paralanguage can become powerful tools for the interpretation of what a patient is conveying.

Perhaps because they are acquired at a very early age, vocal paralinguistic features are the most unconscious aspect of our language use. Not only do we not hear ourselves talk (we are always surprised to hear our voice for the first time on a tape), but we even find it difficult to imitate other speakers simply because we are not consciously aware and in control of paralanguage. Pauses can be perceived as discrete phenomena if pointed out to listeners and contrasted with actual speech. Even speech rate can be easily observed. When it is brought to our attention, we have no trouble recognizing that we perceive someone's speech as fast or slow. But the numerous dimensions that make up the "way we sound" are more difficult to capture, even by skillful listeners. Consequently you must focus attention on such prominent features as pitch, stress, intonation, and voice quality. Obviously this approach does not do justice to the richness of paralinguistic nuances; it will, however, enable you to become aware of inter- and intraspeaker differences, which is the main goal. Since higher pitch and stress normally coincide in English, I will only separate them when they are used in unexpected patterns and convey special meanings.

I will now present a number of examples illustrating the use of vocal paralinguistic features. Read them aloud, and concentrate on the music of speech rather than on the meaning of what is said. If someone else can read them for you, try to observe and describe features such as voice quality, speech rate, intonation, stress, pitch, and disregard what the patients may convey. If you are alone, vary those features as you repeat the examples. Although I realize that this is an artificial task, I believe it will be useful as a teaching device.

In the first example a physician is speaking with a patient he has known for a long time. She is seventy-nine, an upper-middle-class Jewish woman, widowed many years ago. She is carefully dressed, and her hair is very neatly arranged: something she always does when she visits the doctor. She has been ill and is discussing her increasing ability to get around, with which she is justly pleased.

The speakers' use of paralanguage is normal. The animated, almost musical rise and fall of the speech sounds reflects the ease and freedom that mark social conversation among friends:

Well, how are ya?
I'm all right, but I'm still shaky in the legs.
You been out and walkin' around and doin' all those things?
Last time I was here I walked all the way home, my dear. Everybody thought it was crazy. They said, "You walked home from seventy-one—"
Will you do me a big favor and don't tell everybody, or you tell everybody to call me, will you?
Yes. (Snicker).
And how did you do walkin' home?
Well! I walked slowly—
That wasn't so terrible, was it?
No, I walked very—

Who is that "Everybody"?
Oh,—you know, neighbors. But I walked a lot from Seventy-third,
Seventy-second and Second Avenue—to my house. Which is a good
walk, too. Seventy-second and Second Avenue.
Uh-huh.
To my house.
—Y'know,—
But you know with all that walking, Doctor,
Yeah.
—and I take that Valium at night. I don't know those Valium don't
seem to do anything for me. I wake up at two o'clock and I'm finished.

Individual Variation
The next example is of a patient whose speech rate is undeniably fast.
Let us attempt to concentrate on the speech rate alone, in an effort to
isolate it from other paralinguistic features.

This woman is forty-seven years old, American born of Irish parents, an actress. Nothing about her is relaxed. She sits somewhat
forward in her chair, her motions are jerky, and her hands or feet are
always in motion.

Other than that, I only worry about dying of cancer like every one
else. . . . . . What are some of the examinations you should have like,
you know, I have a friend who just had—who's my age who had
the—(I don't know the name of it) but you know, th— the whole—
colon thing 'n all that stuff to make sure everything is really all right.

As native speakers of English, we would all agree on hearing her
that this woman does not have a slow or average speech rate, but
speaks *very* rapidly. At first it might require an effort to limit ourselves
to this observation, because whenever we encounter deviant behavior, our tendency is to assign it some meaning. In the present case
our first reaction would be to say that the woman sounds "nervous"
or "anxious," without realizing that we skipped the observation step
(consciously recognizing the rapidity of her speech) and are "jump-
ing" to conclusions.

The next example also presents a very rapid speech flow:

OK. Bu-ab- as I said about four years ago I had I had dja-thi— and I
smoke. I smoke about—and I don't inhale, I smoke cigars, I maybe
smoke about half a dozen a day.—Very— good cigars that I get from
Mexico, (wheeze) that I get directly from there. Um, no—foreign—
matter or substances in it.—Very cheap but very good. Ah—right
from the tobacco-growing area—

In this case, however, the speaker's rate fluctuates, and as it slows down, his pitch drops. The way the speaker draws out his vowels at the end of the phrases gives his speech an affected dimension. His transitions between phrases are abrupt, resulting in halting, jerky speech and an unusual intonation pattern.

In contrast to the previous examples, the following patient speaks rather slowly:

Actually, I haven't been well for the past—four or five weeks.

What's the matter?

I got a . . . and it was coincidental because the same thing happened to me last year. I had a hemorrhoidal attack but VERY severe.

Mm-hm.

Worse than last year. I went to a proctologist.

Who'd you go to?

I went to ah, Jaxx.

Mm-hm.

(Draws breath) And, he said it was so bad he couldn't even tell me whether—I ha— I would have to have surgery or not. So I got very frightened I had to leave on a trip to—ah, to ah, Europe; a business trip.

Mm-hm.

And, ah, . . . I was in such pain I was in bed for like ten days. I couldn't move, I mean there was no way I could lay. (Clears throat) So finally I uh . . started getting up to walk because I was getting so weak you know.

Mm-hm.

And I started walking weird— to— to, like, kind of, protect it.

Here the overall speech rate is slower than normal, but at times is accelerated. This speaker too draws out syllables, lengthens vowels, creating an impression of some affectation. The patient has a breathy voice quality, a low pitch. Because the speaker lengthens his vowels at the end of phrases without noticeably dropping his pitch, the listener thinks that he has more to say.

Considering speech rate leads us to an interesting observation. When we perceive someone's speech rate as slow or fast, it does not necessarily mean that the speech flow is evenly slow or fast throughout a whole speech segment. A change of rate may occur for a number of reasons, one of which is to highlight some thoughts in contrast to others.

Variations Indicating Meaning Change
The next example exhibits a special pitch/stress pattern, which affects
the meaning of what the patient says.

Now rest your elbows on the table. Elbows. Just remember this is done in the spirit of friendship.
I see. Okay.... Well, let's put it this way, if you can stand it I can.
You—That's MY line!
(Laughter)
That's what I always say to people. But you're absolutely right.
ssss...Je—
Sorry about that.
—sus Christ Almighty—
Okay, Ben.
That's really fuunn. Lets do that agaain.

I mentioned earlier that paralanguage may override the literal
meaning of words: it may mask or even directly contradict the
meaning of words. In this example, because the speaker puts more
than usual stress on unexpected syllables, "That's really FUUNN,"
"Let's do that AGAAIN" (as opposed to the neutral "That's
REALLY fun," "Let's do THAT again") we recognize that the
speaker intends to add meaning that is not contained in the syntax.
The paralanguage contradicts the words and suggests irony: the
patient is not gleefully inviting the doctor to perform another rectal
examination. Clearly the context of the conversation (and our knowledge of the world) also plays an important role in clarifying the
meaning. From what we know of rectal examinations, it is unlikely
that the patient really wants another one.

Variations Due to Cultural Background
The following two examples exhibit paralanguage differences due
mainly to the speakers' cultural backgrounds.

Hello, Doctor. My he— my head.
Yeah.
The other doctor don't help. Eh, yo— No help. Itsa itcha mitcha me.
Mam Mia, my head. You gotta givea me medicine here, f'later, sc—
You mean the shampoo that I gave you last time?
Is it—
—good?

I don't know— I don't know what it is. Y'know— que ser ese, que sere e—
Yeah, I'll give you the lotion that I gave you last time?
(Groan) Oh, Mama Mia, mi— hurtsa me terrible.
Do you remember the lotion I gave you? I'll give you some more.
Well tha— small bottle, I finish with it already.
I'll give you some more. I'll tell—
I'll see you one month, I don't see you.
—him to give you more. I'll tell him to give you more.
You good doctor, you good boy.

This woman's speech is very rapid. Her stress variations and intonation patterns are quite unusual when compared with speakers of English. Furthermore the patient's phonological system is different: she produces sounds in an unusual way. Listeners who have been exposed to Italian immediately recognize it as an Italian accent. Another indication of the patient's foreign origin is the particular syntax and lexicon. In addition to these linguistic differences the speaker's voice has a hoarse quality, probably because she is old.

The next example exhibits a case of paralinguistic variation due to a difference in dialect:

He doesn't want me to do anything for anybody. Don't toek to this one, don't woek here, don't woek there, d— I says, "Hitlaah" I says, "Who the hell da you think you aah?" Scream, I start screaming. Oh, he says he can't take it, he's gotta leave me, he's had enough of me. I says, "Goodbye." What— what are we going to do with him, Dr. Cassell? Nothing. I'm— I says, "You know, Sheldon, I'm still dreaming. I think maybe you'll change but ya never will."

The primary feature revealing this woman's dialect is her phonological system, that is, her pronunciation. Noteworthy in this respect, are her vowels and r-less word endings: HitLAAH (for Hitler), AAH (for are), dAKTAAH (for doctor), WOEK (for walk). The patient also has a changing speech rate: slow at the beginning, then faster, then slow again. She does not drop her pitch at the end of sentences (where it is usually expected), which may be taken by the listener as an indication that she has more to say. The voice quality is hoarse and the pitch low. Because of the combination of paralinguistic features, listeners recognize the speaker as a New Yorker.

Although dialect differences are usually recognized by phonological variations, these are often accompanied by different intonation contours and stress patterns. Difficulty in learning a foreign language or dialect comes when one is unable to distinguish one feature from another and their combinations and, as a result, is unable to reproduce them.

The next patient's mother died recently of scleroderma, and the patient has had recurrent persistent headaches since the death. She is an articulate woman, and she tells us that she finds it difficult to accept her mother's death. But it is her paralanguage that reveals the extent of her emotional involvement: her speech is halting and hesitating, and her voice is slightly hoarse and thin. You can duplicate that change in voice quality by tightening the muscles of your throat. There is little variation in the speaker's overall pattern of intonation. These are the sounds of sadness.

And what's the headache?

. . . . . I think it's that room.

Why should you want that headache not to go away?

. . . . Because it— hh I— I don't know if this makes sense but (sigh) the headache, when I— makes me think of that room and that room was the— last time she was alive! So if you make the headache go away, 'n the room goes away, doesn't it?

Yes, ma'am.

The next example presents a striking contrast. This woman, who now lives in another city, has come back to tell her physician of her good fortune:

Listen, I'm an inspiration to the entire fencing world.—I went to a (laughing) tournament at Christmas. This kid from Brooklyn College fenced about—say, eight, ten years ago, comes a—running up to me, she said, "Jerri, that's terrific! I just heard you were married!" I said "Now let's face it. Why is it terrific? It's terrific because now you think there's hope for you." She said, (whispering) "That's exactly what I thought when I heard it." (Laughter) All my old fencers came back at Christmas and said, "Wow! If you can do it we can do it! A whole new world is open to us!"

The speaker's voice is clear and full, with a rich and varied pattern of intonation. The pitch is relatively high, her speech rate rapid, and the monologue interspersed with laughter. The sound of happiness would be evident, even if the words were obscured.

Let me make the point that the content of a conversation and its paralanguage usually demonstrate the same effect. Occasionally, someone says things that should be sad without the appropriate paralanguage or emits happy sounds with oddly disjunctive content. These distinctions can be obvious or subtle but should not be disregarded.

Paralanguage and Depression

Here are some examples of speech that carry very specific affective information. For the moment, just carefully note them:

And fatigued, huh?
I'm always exhausted. I used to be severely anemic but that— seems—to—have—stopped since the menopause set in. . . . . All my life before that I was quite anemic.
Do you wake up exhausted?
. . Yeah!
Mm-hm.
. . . . It's, uh, . . . I think some of it's emotional—?
Mm-hm.
I had some years of psychotherapy but I'd hate to go back into that.
Mm-hm. —Do you sleep all right?
. . . During the day. (Laughs)
Not at night.
. . . I have trouble FALLING asleep. . . . Once I'm asleep I seem to be all right except if I get the leg cramps or an occasional nightmare.
Mm-hm. —Right. Do you wake up early?
—No. I have a great trouble. All— I've had it all my life—great trouble getting up in the morning but when I have to I do.
Mm-hm.
I set the alarm clock 'nd . . . when I had to be on the job in the morning, I was there.
Mm-hm. How long has this much fatigue gone on for?
Well I've been tired most of my life . . . but, uh—
I mean, right now.
I'd say it's become uh, so that I uh, . . . feel as though I could spend the whole day in bed, for—the last couple months. Two three months perhaps.
Mm-hm. If you spent all day in bed, do you think you'd be any less tired?
I haven't tried it.

This patient's speech rate is slow, her phrasing even. In other words, she has little or no variation in intonation contour; her voice is weak, thin, and breathy. The volume of her voice does not change. Her pausing is unusual in its length and frequency. The pauses are long in relation to the phrases. The pauses have a sharp onset and sharp end, a dead quality. The production of speech seems to require an effort. After this description only one interpretation seems possible: the patient sounds depressed.

Some people may have relatively monotonous contours, slow speech, and so forth, and yet not be depressed. There is no single set of signals that can *infallibly* lead to a correct diagnosis. Paralinguistic cues must be corroborated with information available from the patient's verbal content or other sources. In the case of depression the patient may complain of fatigue, and the present case is a classic description of the fatigue of depression. This fatigue begins immediately on waking up and clears somewhat as the day goes on, or when the person takes part in some kind of satisfying activity—work, and so on. The fatigue of organic disease generally is not present immediately on waking; after a good night's sleep the person feels rested, and fatigue appears after activity and is relieved by a nap. The clinical stakes are very high here, and the physician cannot afford a diagnostic error. The following example is the result of such an error made by a physician-listener who was not alerted to the possibility of depression, despite warning signs in the patient's speech patterns.

I will now present examples of this patient on three different occasions: an early stage of her depression, deeply into her depression, and after her depression.

This woman is sixty-two years old, white, and a widow. Her accent is white Southern Appalachian. Listeners with a really good ear would be able to identify exactly where she grew up, since accents vary in different parts of the same region. Her recent years have been marked by sadness since her husband's death. Her son has had considerable difficulty and his daughter, her favorite granddaughter, was found dead in a hotel room within the year. She is obese and has hypertension and diabetes.

... if I could keep my pressure down, but everything has happened that could possibly happen, even a leak—come pourin' down ... I mean, i ... everything has happened that—could possibly happen even w— with tragedy ... i-It's happened. A leak come pouring down through the ceiling. ... You know, in the bedroom. ... I-It's—

—*That doesn't help your hypertension, huh?*

No it certainly didn't when you didn't know where it was goin' it just happened that I got the Super right fast to stop it. Y'know?
Mm-hm.
And he's not that easy got, but I found him. . . . And if I name all the things, you wouldn't wonder why it's up.

In this first segment the patient's speech is slow, halting, and hesitant; her pausing is somewhat unusual; her voice lacks normal strength and fullness. Although the patient stresses individual words, her overall intonation pattern is limited, as well as her volume and pitch range. Naturally this combination of features is accompanied by the patient's individual voice quality and phonological system. Now for the second example:

Mm-hm. Short of breath?
A small amount.
When will that show itself, Mary?
. . . . . . It's just that I can hardly make it.
How'd you get here today?
On the train.
How'd you get up the steps?
I had to walk that.
Mm-hm. How long— how many times did you stop coming up those steps? . . . Did you have to stop at all or did you just walk slow?
I just walked slow. . . . . Well, on the landing I waited. You know I didn't rush up. . . . I had to go slow.
Now, what slows you down, Mary?
. . . Just weakness.
Weakness. Not your breathing? Your breathing's okay? That's not what's slowing you down?
I— It's just that I can't . . .
Can't what?
—Can't really make it.
Mm-hm. Do you sleep at night?
. . . . . . Pretty good. . . . . Fairly good.
Are you urinating a lot?
. . . Fairly.
Do you have to get up at night to urinate?
. . . Some times.
Mm-hm. Is your appetite good?

There was never wrong with that but it's not eating. Every time I try to lose weight, this— I get weak.

Well, is that why you're weak now; because you're trying to lose weight?

Well I don't know what else. You know . . . . . . I . . I just can't guess because I don't know.

In the preceding segment, taped nine months later, the same paralinguistic pattern prevails, but it is much more accentuated by now: her voice is even weaker, more thin and breathy. A listener has no trouble hearing that the patient produces speech only with great effort. As a result she limits her talk to answering the doctor's questions with isolated utterances.

As embarrassing as it is to admit it, I am her physician. I kept questioning her to find out what was causing her weakness. I listened carefully to what she said, but not to how she said it. In those days I simply did not know about the paralanguage characteristics of depression. In retrospect of course the content should also have alerted me to her obvious full-blown depression. She had a stroke two months later, and while she was in the hospital, I finally recognized her depression. It was successfully treated.

The next segment was recorded a number of months later. I purposely introduced topics similar to those on the previous tape, for the sake of contrasting normal with depressed speech:

Now, tell me again, ah, about coming here. You ha— you ha— a-a— about coming up the subway steps. It's always a problem, you said?

It's a problem because I have to step just one little step at a time and have to pull my— you know, I can't come up like I used to.

Mm-hm. Do you get short of breath comin' up?

No. (Slight laugh)

Uh-huh. And is it hard for you or just because of the we— I mean tell me more about it.

Well, my weight is not good—

Uh-huh.

—for comin' up them steps.

Mm-hm, mm-hm. And how are things at the building?

Well, uh— (laughs and clears throat) last year I couldn' a stood what I had this year on account a th— so much snow and the salt 'n—

Mm-hm.

(Clears throat) Now it changed from salt to (cough) excuse me, oils, oil spill. Now they're trackin' it in.

In this postdepression segment the patient's speech has regained its strength. It has fuller, richer intonation contours, a broader range of vocal contrasts, and short pauses. Her speech rate is still slow and her voice hoarse, but again, these seem related to her individual speech characteristics. She has difficulty with pronunciation as the result of a stroke, but it is clear that she is no longer depressed.

The characteristic features of the speech of depressed patients appear to be closely related to the fact that their speech production requires an extraordinary effort. Their breath intake and supply do not seem to provide sufficient air to allow a normal and full flow of sounds. As a measure of economy their pausing increases, their speech rate drops, their intonation contours are limited and so is their verbal output. In short, their symptoms are manifested in their speech.

The case of this woman should make it clear that knowledge of paralanguage, and other aspects of language use, are important additions to a physician's store of clinically useful tools.

As with all other clinical skills considerable practice is required before you will be able to hear paralinguistic features as distinct entities. It is my hope that you will begin to hear the spoken language as you have never heard it before.

References

Allport, G. W., and H. Cantrill. Judging personality from voice. *J. Soc. Psychol.* 1934, 5, 37.

Brown, B. L., W. J. Strong, and A. C. Rencher. Fifty-four voices from two: the effects of simultaneous manipulations of rate, mean fundamental frequency and variance of fundamental frequency on ratings of personality from speech. *Acoust. Soc. Am. J.* 1974, 55, 2, 313–318.

Brown, B. L., W. J. Strong, and A. C. Rencher. Perceptions of personality from speech: effects of manipulation of acoustical parameters. *Acoust. Soc. Am. J.* 1973, 54, 29–35.

Brown B., and W. E. Lambert. A cross-cultural study of social status markers in speech. *Canadian J. Behavioral Science*, 1976, 8, (1), 39–55.

Davitz, J. R. *The communication of emotional meaning*. New York: William Alanson White Institute.

Davitz, J. R. The communication of feelings by content free speech. *J. Communication*, 1959, 9, 6–13.

Eldred, S. H., and D. B. Price. A linguistic evaluation of feeling states in psychotherapy. *Psychiatry*, 1958, 21, 115–121.

Fay, P. J., and W. C. Middleton. The ability to judge sociability from the voice as trasmitted over a public address system. *J. Soc. Psychol.* 1944, 13, 303.

Goldman-Eisler, F. *Psycholinguistic experiments in spontaneous speech*. New York: Academic Press, 1968.

Hunt, R. G., and T. K. Lin. Accuracy of judgements of personal attributes from speech. *J. Pers. Soc. Psychol.* 1967, 6, 450.

Maclay, H., and C. E. Osgood. Hesitation phenomena in spontaneous English speech. *Word*, 1959, 15, 19–44.

Mahl, G. F. Disturbances in the patient's speech as a function of anxiety. In *Trends in Content Analysis*. Ed. by I. Pool. Urbana: Univ. of Illinois, 1959.

Mahl, G. F. Disturbances and silences in the patient's speech in psychotherapy. *J. Abnom. Soc. Psychol.* 1956, 53, 1–15.

Mahl, G. F., and G. Schulze. Psychological research in the extralinguistic area. In *Approaches to Semiotics*. Ed. by Th. Sebeok, A. Hayes, and M. C. Bateson. The Hague: Mouton, 1964, pp. 51–123.

Pope, B., T. Blass, A. W. Siegman, and J. Raher. Anxiety and depression in speech. *J. Consult. Psych.* 1970, 35, 128–133.

Williams, C. E., and K. N. Stevens. Emotions and speech: some acoustical correlates. *Acoust. Soc. Am. J.* 1972, 52, 1238–1249.

2

The Interior World of Language:
What You Say Is Who You Are

When we think about what language "is," we usually consider it to be a system of symbols which "stands for" objects (tangible and intangible), relations, and events in the world. Equally, language can describe imaginary objects, fantasy relations, and dream events. Clearly, then, the use of language is not confined to the real (shared) world. Because language can be used in diverse ways, an individual's language use does more than describe worlds real and imaginary; it characterizes the *language user* as well. Attention to word choice, syntax, as well as paralinguistic cues such as pause, pitch, voice color, and speech rate can reward the careful listener with a great deal of information about speakers' worlds and their relation to them— about their beliefs and what is feared, celebrated, denied, valued (or disvalued), and adored. Learning to listen skillfully to the patient and to interpret judiciously what is said can be as critical a diagnostic tool as learning to hear and interpret heart sounds. This is a major focus of this chapter.

This chapter also concerns the *therapeutic* significance of language. By means of language we not only describe reality, we actually *appropriate* it; that is, we make it "real" to ourselves. And this appropriation may be—and usually is—highly individual. Whereas one sibling may think of her mother as "being crippled," another describes her as "having a slight limp." Similarly an illness can be "dreadful," "horrible," or only "annoying"; it may even be "challenging," or even "enlightening." Language can not only describe reality, it can create it. This is the genius of language, and its therapeutic significance for the physician. It can be used in the clinical setting either carefully and therapeutically, or else without thought, and often to the patient's detriment.

We begin, then, by looking at words. Not, however, words in isolation but words as they reflect the kinds of language use— language groupings. Only at this level of complexity will language begin to reveal the speaker in any depth. This approach should not be unfamiliar, since understanding "objective" physical processes requires such an approach as well. Years ago, in a hematology course, my instructor banged the blackboard for attention. Once too often a student had asked the instructor to peer through the microscope, asking "What is that cell?" "You always want to know what 'that cell' is solely by looking at the isolated cell. If you want to know what a cell is and what it means, don't just look at it—see the company it keeps!" So it is with the meaning of spoken language. You must learn to hear not only individual words, but the *kinds* of nouns, adjectives, verbs, adverbs, and pronouns speakers use as well as the syntax employed to put them together. You are always trying to find out how speakers view *themselves* in relation to what they are speaking about— as well as what they are speaking!

Adjectives

Adjectives are words that modify nouns. To listen to adjectives is to hear some of the connotative meanings of the nouns: what things denoted by the noun mean to the speaker. Here are some examples.

This woman is speaking to the surgeon who resected her carcinoma of the colon.

Hello! How are you.

Well, that's— that's a good question. As far as your work, I think I'm getting along all right. I had a stomach upset for the first time in months. I went to a couple of parties, stupidly forgot and ate all s— all ridiculous things, and I had a terrible— terrible movement and then terrible diarrhhea. This was Tuesday. So I— I took a little Lowe—Lomotil and it stopped it, but I haven't, um, taken any mineral oil because I'm afraid of starting up again.

Mm-hm.

But this was my first upset, but I did a very stupid thing. I have been careful of my diet since I had my surgery—

Righ. Okay—

But I haven't had any pains or aches or— as far as it's concerned.

This, ah, diarrhea business, has stopped now?

Oh, completely.

She had "terrible movements" and "terrible diarrhea." We do not know what about the bowel movement was "terrible," and even if we did know we might not think they were "terrible." But there must be something that is part of its meaning to her besides the general definition—frequent loose stools—to make that diarrhea "terrible." She also said "I did eat some very stupid things." What made these (foodstuff) things "stupid" to eat? A woman concerned about her recently operated bowels might think Southern fried chicken and corn-on-the-cob "stupid." A hot Indian curry merits the same adjective. Both dishes can also be called (variously) delicious, exciting, heartwarming, exotic. There is something contained within the meaning of these foods that is unwise for delicate bowels and which (or I could not use them as examples) is known to many.

Foods also *do* things: an apple a day keeps the doctor away, raw oysters are an aphrodisiac. And what foods do is part of their meaning. This begins to show us how inclusive the meanings of words can be.

The next example will advance the argument.

Ah, I went to see him on the Tuesday after last Saturday when it happened; he examined me and said, "Aha! A cyst on your ovary." *Mm-hm.*
Which scared the hell out of me to begin with! But he is a very reasonable man, a reassuring man, and not a belittling man.

See what kind of a doctor he is: reassuring, and reasonable, and not belittling. But in what context? The doctor has found an ovarian cyst, and the news of the finding scared the patient. This is not precisely what the patient said; rather, "he said, aha! a cyst on your ovary," and that was what scared "hell" out of her. Is he a doctor who tells patients about ovarian cysts in order to scare them? No, he is a "reasonable," "reassuring," and "not belittling" doctor. Surely such a doctor does not tell about ovarian cysts in order to frighten.

On hearing this tape, a medical student said, "I know what she means: I had a dentist, every time he found a cavity he acted like he'd scored!" (A word of caution: we cannot know precisely what the patient meant, especially from a few phrases quoted out of context. This discussion assumes that the entire conversation supports the conclusion. In actual practice the listener might use this interpretation as an hypotheses and seek more information to support or negate the conclusion.)

In listening, the student used his own experiential knowledge of dentists as the interpretor of this patient's meaning. But can we, merely hearing her words, come to some conclusion about how she pictures herself in relation to the events being recounted. The patient says that her first assumption about doctors who tell about ovarian cysts is that doctors frighten and belittle. This is odd. It is not *my* first assumption, although I know what she means. But in addition to frightening, doctors also "belittle." This usage is less common. Her words do not imply that doctors *intend* to frighten and belittle.

Why do I say this is her first assumption? Because the patient says, "He said it was an ovarian cyst, which scared hell out of me, *but* he is a reassuring, etc." The word *but* implies he is *X rather than Y*. The *Y* is unspoken. (In chapter 3 I shall discuss the logical operations performed by words like "but," "if," and "or.")

If this patient believes that doctors belittle their patients, though she thinks that you, her doctor, do not, it matters little whether you do. She will view everything you say in the light of this suspicion, and it will take a long time for your reasonable, reassuring, and nonbelittling behavior to replace the opposite in the meaning she attaches to the word "physician." Further, if this patient believes that doctors might be frightening and belittling, then she must see herself as someone who can be belittled and frightened. Or, to put it simply, her description of what doctors do suggests that she herself is fearful and unconfident. Remember, when people describe the world, they must *inevitably* describe themselves in relation to that world.

You may wonder at the amount of interpretation given this phrase. To be believable, such interpretation requires the assumption that speakers say precisely what they mean, that words mean what they say, and that word choice is not random or haphazard. As the Mad Hatter says in *Alice in Wonderland*, "I say what I mean, and I mean what I say." Speakers do, indeed, say what they mean. A few months of attentive listening will remove any doubts. To the extent that she was able to use words to express her meanings, this patient said what she meant.

What *is* impossible to believe is that any listener can interpret to this degree as conversation proceeds. Not only were the phrases finished in about ten seconds, but also conversation continued, drawing attention from further interpretation. Attentive listeners develop an ability to hear as talk goes on but, at the same time, keep the last few phrases in active memory—like those intensive-care monitors that display instantaneous data but also keep the information in memory for a few seconds so that it can be "frozen" and examined. This facility allows the listener to react instantly to what is said, as well as to interpret.

In the conversation we have been discussing, as you listened, you would form a notion of four distinctly separate but related things: you would hear her opinion of doctors in general; you would hear her opinion of her own doctor; and at the same time, you would hear her opinion telling you about her; and you would hear the actual events unfolding in the narration. This skill, as well as the necessary ability to remember precisely what the patient said and how, is acquired with time. It is no more complex than the ability to listen with the stethescope to first one then the other heart sound, or one part of the cardiac cycle at a time.

This consideration of adjectives has shown how much larger is the meaning of nouns like "diarrhea," "food," or "doctor" than is generally considered. The dictionary or denotative meaning is only the skeleton of meaning these words can have.

Adjectives do something else. They also express the "value" aspects of nouns, the good and badness of the meanings in all the various dimensions in which good and bad can be expressed: from the "powdery (good) snow" for skiers to the "fast (bad) food" for gourmets. This "good" and "bad" becomes part of the thought expressed by the noun phrase, "a reassuring and not belittling man." Evaluating attitudes about feelings and about things is part of thinking about them.

Adjectives are basically descriptive terms, and an accurate description of symptoms is of vital importance to physicians. Therefore careful listening to this aspect of adjectival function is a way of establishing vital diagnostic clues.

Do you have difficulty breathing or anything?
Um, I have this—sort of a smothery little feeling.
—Smothery inside, yeah.

What is the difficulty with the patient's breathing? "A sort of smothery little feeling."

Notice first that it is NOT a "smothering feeling," that is, a feeling as though she were about to smother. Rather, the feeling shares characteristics with smothering: "sort of smothery." Both "sort of" and the "ery" ending diminish smothering. Smothering is a major sensation. Hers is a "little" feeling.

Although patients who are not articulate may have to be offered descriptive word choices (carefully, in order to avoid "putting words in their mouths"), generally very accurate descriptions of symptoms can be achieved; these often correlate with pathophysiology within high confidence limits. Patience, careful listening, and experience sufficient to recognize how pathophysiology expresses itself in symptoms are required. For example, the intense, gripping, squeezing, substernal pain of esophageal spasm—so often confused with angina pectoris—is an example of a symptom which, if carefully elicited, tells one much about how the esophagus functions (and dysfunctions), and even about its nerve supply. Careful listening in that setting may also avoid a hospital admission.

In this next example a patient is reacting to her weight—and telling us about herself.

Is that your weight over there?
Yeah, and it's honest. And it's bad. But I'm— not going to fight it anymore. You look marvelously slender, but I— I just— I can't do it.
You can't do it, hmm?
Nah.
All right.
The thin-thing-within-me just won't come out 'cause I won't let it.

This patient is obviously heavy, by *her standards*. We do not know how heavy she actually is, because sometimes ballet dancers who are as big around as your little finger make similar remarks. In this country, as Mrs. Paley is said to have said, you can't be too thin or too rich.

When the patient says the weight is "bad," the implication is that *she* is bad. All of us have heard this kind of conversation in which people describe themselves by means of a part of themselves. Her weight on the scale is also "honest," implying that one might be tempted to set the scale lighter. I am sure there is a "thin thing within her," and experience also tell us it never will come out. Pity.

Such "small talk" about weight is very common and often revealing, especially if the physician can avoid getting caught up in the patient's emotional games about weight.

Verbs

Verbs are words of action, and they place the speaker in relationship to objects and events. Thus, they may tell us how the speaker sees himself, or herself, in relation to these objects or events:

And, uh, Jerry did an EKG, and he stuck me right into the hospital.

He was "stuck right in the hospital!" The patient could have said "and then Jerry admitted me to the hospital," or "so I went to the hospital," and "so I dived right into . . ." or "Jerry asked me to go, so I went to the hospital."

Were you in the Intensive Care Unit? The Cardiac Intensive Care Unit?
Ah, there wasn't any room there. But they had me hooked up to other machines.
How fortunate—

He was "hooked up" to all the machines. He could have been "connected to," or "monitored by," or "the machines were all connected to me," or "watched over by all the machines."

If we were to ask Jerry about the same events, he might have said "Then I admitted him to the hospital. There were no CCU beds so I had him monitored on the floor." The feeling tone of these verbs is much more neutral than the patient's usage. He was "stuck in . . ." like a bag of laundry. Passive in the hospital, and passively connected to machines. It will be no surprise that, later in the conversation, the patient expressed overt resentment at what was, to him, an unnecessary hospitalization. No one likes to be passive in such situations. Illness removes control from patients' volitions sufficiently without, as they see it, doctors adding to this lack of control.

The "facts" are that the patient was in the doctor's office and subsequently, in the hospital. But language—verbs in this instance—can redefine reality in terms of the speaker: diarrhea (frequent loose stools) becomes "terrible"; the doctor is no longer merely a six-foot person who weights 165 pounds, but "marvelously slender." What an advantage over the real world where a "rose is a rose is a rose."

In the universe of spoken language the world can be changed, and changed, and changed again to fit the needs of the speaker. The speaker's relationship to that world can be expressed in verbs like "stuck," "run," "jump," "break." The speaker can do the acting on or be acted on. Verbs of state are different: to "think," "need," "want," "know." Various emotions can be expressed through verbs of action and through verbs of state. "Talk" and "persuade" are both active, but "persuade" carries more charge, as does "cajole" and "wheedle." "Induce" and "convince" are milder verbs, describing the same process as "persuade." "Love" is a verb of state, as is "care," but they have quite different emotional loading.

The plasticity of the world of language in relation to the real world is developed by syntax. Each verb can be used in more than one way. When children are learning to talk, they construct only simple declarative sentences such as, "I hit the ball." If they are given a sentence like "The truck was hit by the car" to act out, they will have the truck hit the car. With increasing age comes increasing sophistication and the ability to construct complex sentences that allow reality to be further shaped through language. Verbs express what the speaker witnesses, does, and endures and hence express the speakers's *world*.

Adverbs

Adverbs modify verbs, as adjectives modify nouns, to extend the range of possible meanings.

And I was in torture. Absolute torture. My arm was a wing—it hung. Lifelessly. Painfully.

The broken arm did not just hang. It "hung lifelessly." And yet not devoid of life, because it also hung "painfully." This is the same woman with the "thin thing within her." She achieves this dramatic quality by a richness of word usage, in this instance, by modifying the verb "to hang" with both "lifelessly" and "painfully."

Hello! How are you.
Well, that's— that's a good question. As far as your work, I think I'm getting along all right. I had a stomach upset for the first time in months. I went to a couple of parties, stupidly forgot and ate all s— all ridiculous things, and I had a terrible— terrible movement and then terrible diarhhea. This was Tuesday. So I— I took a little Lowe— Lomotil and it stopped it, but I haven't, um, taken any mineral oil because I'm afraid of starting up again.
Mm-hm
But this was my first upset, but I did a very stupid thing. I have been careful of my diet since I had my surgery—

This is the patient who not only eats "ridiculous things" but also modifies the verb "to forget" with "stupidly." "Stupidly" forgetting is far stronger than simply to forget. This is an active process, revealing her self-blame. She could have "carelessly" forgotten, "absent-mindedly" forgotten, or "simply" forgotten. Each adverb changes the nature of the act of forgetting by involving the patient more or less actively in it. Although we cannot read the "little black box" of the patient's mind, we can read her words. Thus we know from her choice of words that a volitional "her" is involved and that she holds herself accountable, even to the point of self-denigration, for forgetting. Since, as her doctor, I want to know about that person, I note her use of descriptive terms as *self*-description. Keep in mind that this self-description occurs when she is talking to me (her doctor) and that in conversation with another person, she might use different language.

Speakers' Choice of Words

I'm not sure that it's connected, so I'll give you both— both ends of it. We were in Europe, we were schlepping around baggage.

Just as speakers have characteristic paralanguage, they have idiosyncratic, and even culturally characteristic, word choice. One patient says, "We were shlepping that baggage all over Europe." Another says, "We were lugging that baggage all over Europe." Both verbs, "to schlep and "to lug," denote more than ordinary effort. The speaker who uses the word "schlep," which comes from Yiddish, is probably Jewish, or from New York City.

Some speakers use a much more brightly colored palette of words than others. Things are "terrible," "marvelous," "wonderful," "smashing," "fantastic." They "schlep" baggage, "gobble up" a book, are "overwhelmed" by London. No pastels for these people. Such vocabularies are often called theatrical. For others, things are "nice," "lovely," "unpleasant," "touching." Others "browse" in the same book, "carry" their baggage, and "enjoy" London. The importance to the attentive physician of this common observation is that symptoms of illness are also described using that person's characteristic palette of words. A pain, "excruciating" to one patient might be "unpleasant" to another. Every practitioner knows that it is easier to take telephone calls from one's own patient than from the patient of another physician. You know much better what your own patient means than when listening to a stranger, because you have become acclimated to his or her manner of speech, registering, usually below awareness, the word choice, syntax, and paralanguage (among other personal characteristics). Thus you have a standard, tacit or acknowledged, against which to measure current complaints. The sociologist, Mark Zborowski in his book *People in Pain*, documented the fact that patients from different ethnic backgrounds react differently to pain. If this is true, and we all know it is, how do doctors ever make a diagnosis? How can we distinguish between a "terrible" (Jewish) pain and an "annoying" (Irish) pain?

Young physicians frequently make errors based on those different usages. If the patient says "terrible," they think it means the same as they, the doctors, would mean by "terrible." When the pain turns out to have been of more benign origins, the physician may feel cheated, as though the patient lied. The reverse also holds. When the patient's "annoying" pain comes from a very serious source, the unpracticed physician says, aggrieved, "The patient never told me." This kind of experience may be one source of the very common attitude among medical students, interns, and residents that patients do not tell the truth. It is absolutely essential that the meaning the doctor (listener) attaches to descriptive language not be confused with the patient's meaning.

How is the listener to solve this vital problem? By listening to the vocabulary the speaker employs in the remainder of a conversation. When word choice is extreme and colorful for everything else, so, too, will it be for pain, shortness of breath, diarrhea. Generally, muted speakers will also understate their symptoms.

The conversation may not go on long enough, however, to provide clues to the patients' characteristic mode of speech. I have learned two ways of dealing with this. When I first meet a new patient, even in an emergency room, much of my early conversation sounds like small talk, pleasantries to pass the time. Although I value politeness, this is not my prime motivation. I am trying to get the patient to talk, so that I can hear how he or she uses words, syntax, and paralanguage, in order to have a standard against which to compare the description of symptoms. Further, in taking the past history or review of systems, I look for some previous experience with pain against which to measure the patient's words. "Have you ever had a pain like this?" "Just last week—terrible, almost unendurable—I caught my finger in a zipper—it must have lasted ten minutes—simply agonizing." I think you may safely tell the surgeon to go home, this patient will probably survive.

On the other hand: "Have you ever had a pain like this?" "No, this is really quite uncomfortable." "When did you last see a physician?" "About ten years ago." "Any serious accidents, or break any bones?" "Well, yes. Fractured my left leg in a camping accident—had to walk eighteen miles after that to get help, what an annoyance." Tell the surgeon to stick around.

This is not to suggest that people who exaggerate never have pain, they most assuredly do. Nor do I mean to imply that phlegmatic people cannot be hypochondriachal, they most certainly can. Nevertheless, their language in both instances will be a more reliable indicator, be more specific and sensitive, than many other diagnostic tools.

A word of caution. A pain may be designated "terrible" by the most stoical if the pain has acquired terrible significance. If the patient believes with all his or her heart that the pain represents cancer of the pancreas, in a family in which all have died awful deaths from cancer of the pancreas, then the pain will acquire the language appropriate to its meaning, not to its actual sensory magnitude. Here, one can be misled. But the problem is solved by asking appropriate questions.

In our professional lives we usually treat patients from the same culture as our own. As a result culture and language are automatically taken into account. Because we and our patients have the same values, we *do* know what they mean when they say something or do something, and we know what illness, hospitals, and paralysis mean to the patients because, generally speaking, they mean the same to us. Thus we can get away with not being an attentive listener, because all we have to do is listen to ourselves and most often we know what the patient means. For those of us who train in hospitals where the patients' backgrounds may diverge radically from our own, the assumptions of shared meanings do not suffice. It is in such settings that the patients' different language practices—word usage, syntax, and paralanguage—are frequently brushed aside, or looked down on. It *is* disconcerting to speak to a Greek who shakes his head no and means yes! But, one learns.

In this era it is not necessary to argue in favor of crosscultural understanding; everybody knows its importance. What is not so obvious is that *all* communication shares the same fundamental problems as crosscultural communication. Remember you are already dealing with two translators in any conversation: the patient's understanding of your meaning, and your understanding of his or hers.

Changing the World by Changing the Words

I began this chapter by stating that the language a person uses in speaking about objects, people, or events tells the listener not only about these matters but also about what kind of a person the speaker is. That is because, in describing these subjects, the speaker is in some sense describing his or her relationship to them or beliefs about them. The mind uses the symbols that make up language to construct a transliteration from the outside world of reality to the inside world of symbols.

The semantic world differs from the real world in a number of respects, but one that is particularly important has to do with valuing. Language confers value on virtually everything and every relationship it describes. Nothing has value in and of itself. There are no "tall" or "short" trees. True, there are trees of 100 feet and trees of 10 feet, but "tall" and "short" are human concepts. So are "fat" and "thin." Because attitudes inevitably become associated with such adjectives, so that, say, tall trees become more desirable than short trees, the word "tall" in conjunction with trees confers value. The world of language then is a world of values. And what we value helps shape each of us as individuals. Values also partially define a culture.

Even if you agree with these statements, you may wonder about their relevance to clinical medicine. Their applicability comes from recognition of the advantage possessed by the world of language over the real world. In the symbolic world of language reality can be manipulated. Threats can be mitigated. They can also be magnified. Objects, relationships, and events can be changed, enlarged, reduced, obliterated, simply by changing the words that describe them. The potential use in clinical medicine is clear: doctors can use the spoken word to change the perception of reality for patients! An anthropologist told me once of a terror-filled nighttime ride through the African bush. One of the members of the group had been bitten by a snake that another knew to be poisonous. They killed the snake, applied first aid, and headed for the nearest doctor, miles away. As the ride progressed, the injured person developed increasingly severe symptoms of venom poisoning. The others panicked, and by the time they reached the hospital, the whole group was hysterical. The doctor looked at the snake and said, "that snake is not poisonous." The "patient," when finally convinced, recovered rapidly, and everyone was very chagrined. The doctor changed reality by those few words. You may object that the doctor did not *change* reality but merely confirmed it. The doctor changed *their* reality, which was that the snake was poisonous and, unless aid was quickly reached, the man would die. That was their reality, and they acted on it. The patient's symptoms may have been hysterical, but a death from the Land Rover going into a ravine, a very possible event, would not have been hysterical—and *their* reality had been created by the words "the snake is poisonous."

Taboo subjects provide another example. Patients avoid certain subjects or words, speaking as though the associated event, organ, or symptom does not exist:

I was fine until 1968.
You were fine until '68. What happened in 1968?
I got another— another attack.
You got another attack of— of breathlessness?
Yeah . . . . Same thing.
What were you doing that time?
Electrical industry. The same thing. I was— in '68 I was in, ah,
I mean, what were ya— were you going down some stairs, or walking, or doing something active, or lying in bed?
I was in action.
Huh?
(Loud whisper) Sex!
Oh! I see.
All right?
Okay.

This patient is giving the history of his heart attack. Asked about his activity at the time of the episode, he tries at first to avoid answering, then switches to a euphemism. Euphemisms are nice words for subjects that are being avoided: "bathroom tissue" instead of "toilet paper." The patient uses the word "action" to stand for having intercourse. When pressed, he says "sex"—but in a loud whisper. Sometimes we even say that an action is unspeakable, as though to say it is to be injured by the word itself. This next patient is discussing the choice of operation for a breast malignancy:

What happens if, for instance, everything's cleaned out and yet, below the below the below is also—infected—?

What is "below the below the below"? In the world of language, things are not true unless they are said. (And in an odd way things may indeed be not true until said, in the sense that until people begin to act on the stated knowledge, the whole truth is not out.) I remember a woman protecting her just-deceased father from the doctor, saying "I won't let you pronounce him dead!" It is as though the father will not be dead unless pronounced. Such a mechanism may have limited utility, as this example illustrates. But when saying something removes all doubt, so long as the truth remains unspoken, reality can be kept at bay. Thus before the confession of infidelity the loved one could be considered (in the inner world which is where we all really live) *not* to have been unfaithful. You may say of the case, "That is denial," of the other, "That is lying." The fact remains that we do not act on the basis of reality, but on our conception of it. Our conception of reality is frequently conveyed, in whole or part, by language.

Of course the relationship of language to reality has another face. When something is *not* spoken it can remain within, if only as a suspicion to become in fears and fantasies larger than reality. The unspoken can overwhelm us. But once it is uttered, we have become larger than it. As we shall see, this allows the doctor to use words like "cancer," "death," "blindness," "schizophrenia," in conversation and, by so doing, relieve the patient's fears. By saying the words, the doctor brings out the concepts for which the words stand, showing that these concepts, which were previously inside terrorizing the patient, are smaller than the doctor. Otherwise, the doctor would have been unable to say the words. Similarly, euphemisms, like an "active" tumor or "mitoses," usually do not fool the patient but, instead, demonstrate that the doctor is afraid of the disease, object, or event. Judging by how many years it took me to learn to say "death," "dying," "dead," in conversations with patients and their families, the belief that fear of the word is fear of the thing is justified.

It is important for you to recognize that a similar mechanism for avoiding painful reality is operating when a patient switches to generalities or abstractions: "Have you been wheezing lately?" "Isn't that what asthmatics do?" "Yes, but have you been wheezing?" "Well, this is the pollen season, so I suppose I should be having trouble ..." When you manage to nail the patient down to specifics, you almost always find that the details are unpleasant and a cause of alarm for the patient, hence the attempt at avoidance.

The next example demonstrates a fascinating way in which the patient's language gives a glimpse into her perception of reality.

Yes—

What does one do to remove a cyst on an ovary.

Remove it or look at it?

No-no. R-r-r-emove it. He said that if it's still there after his— after his—

He must operate on you.

Isn't that funny. But one has an image of injecting the vagina w-w-with a— no, with the, with the necessary equipment, and then one blows up by becoming pregnant. Is that the same— the same feeling that I am having now, that if one sticks anything at all into what is an impervious breast, one becomes blown up and what does one make?

This is the same patient as "below the below," and the monologue is odd. Whose breast is she discussing? "*One's* breast." Who is "one?" Is "one's breast" the same as "my breast?"

The following example makes two important points. The first is that technical language can also be a means to avoid contact with an intrusive reality. Such language is often employed to keep "what we know" at a distance from "what we feel" and so can readily be usurped when a subject is anxiety provoking. The second point, perhaps more important, is how the speaker's choice of pronouns can be employed to manipulate reality.

I was teaching a course on interviewing, and a patient was brought from the floors to be interviewed by another physician who did not know her. When the interviewer said, "What brought you to the hospital?" the patient answered, "Acute lymphoblastic leukemia." That finished the interviewer; he never regained control of the demonstration. The rest of us did not recover from it either. The patient proceeded to give the class a lecture on her inevitably fatal disease. How could she do that? I played and replayed the tape recording of the interview, trying to hear the means by which she could so calmly discuss what would soon kill her. It certainly did not seem like denial, at least not as I knew it. Here is a brief portion of her conversation:

It seems like, ah, they feel that people that have leukemia have been tired all their life or suffering with anemia or something similar, which was not the case whatsoever. I seemed healthy for forty-four and a half years and, ah, I would say that this is another thing no one seems to know— whether you have this long before it shows up, or whether you just got it and, ah, it shows.

Ah, you say you felt tired?

After I quit smoking.

Note that the symptoms of leukemia—fatigue, anemia, "or something similar"—belong to "people who have leukemia," not to this patient. To her belongs health—"I seemed healthy for forty-four and a half years...." Note also "*You* have this long before it shows up, or whether *you* just got it." Who is "you"? Why is the pronoun "I" not employed by her? She is, after all, talking about herself. What does the word "it" refer to? This patient has managed, by her choice of pronouns (and technical language) to *depersonalize* her own illness!

An interesting aspect of this is how long it took me to hear the phenomenon originally. I played the tape again and again. After realizing what was going on, I went over another transcript from a dying patient. I was sure that I would see the shift of pronouns from personal to impersonal when death or illness was discussed. I searched the transcript but could not find the shift. It had to be there! Again I read but could not find it. It was the third reading before I could identify the words that were under my eyes all the time. This way of handling difficult or painful material is so common that it is almost invisible (or inaudible). I was unaware that this phenomenon had been described a number of years earlier by several authors and discussed, in 1969, by David Bakan in his book, *Death, Pain and Suffering*.

Here is another example (with the impersonal pronouns capitalized):

But there— uh, it came on me, uh, just woke up in the middle of the night, and I thought I was havin' a stroke or somethin'—that's the way it comes on. And YOU lose YOUR sense of balance and YOU vomit, and it's a terrible-YOU don't know what's the matter with YOU. YOU have no pain, but there's somethin' wrong. Then when that passes away then YOU'RE lucky if YOU don't have it, like every couple years. See, a lot of peoples have it comin'— comes back on them, but I may never have another attack.

Once again the symptoms belong to the impersonal "you." But "no further attacks" belong to "I." (She is speaking of Meniere's Syndrome.) You may wonder why she can say "I thought I was having a stroke, or something"—perhaps because she did *not* in fact have a stroke or perhaps because no language clue is invariably accurate.

Thus the world of language has another advantage over the real world: the integrity of self can be protected by constructing a depersonalized self, literally a self from which the speaker's person has been withdrawn. And on this depersonalized entity, variously called "you," "one," or not identified at all, can fall the slings and arrows of outrageous fortune.

Contrast these next two examples:

I, ah, sleep on my stomach a lot.
Mm-hm.

And, ah, I don't know if it's imagination or all the hubbub about it, I just felt that my breasts were hurting a little bit.

If you see something on a mammogram, does that mean you have to have the breast removed?

No.

In the first example, the patient speaks of "my breasts." In the second example, it is "the breast." Women do not speak about their breast as "*the* breast." They almost invariably say "my breast." They may speak of "the nipple" but they say "my breast," until something happens to it or it is endangered, at which time it becomes "the breast." When women have mastectomies, the removed breast is referred to as "the breast," which seems quite natural. However, the remaining normal breast is often then also referred to as "the breast." As the months pass after operation, it becomes "my breast."

Two more examples:

Well, two things have been bugging me for a long time, and I have looked into it. It's this hissing sound in my ear which I— I've gone to ear doctors. And I've had floating spots in my eyes, and I've seen my eye doctor.

This is the usual way in which people refer to their eyes, ears, arms, and legs, but in the next example:

Now—

What's the matter there?

I don't know. I get headaches when I get up in the morning and I feel as if I was drunk, and it seems—

Mm-hm.

It sort of—effects this part across THE eyes here.

"The eyes" is unusual. All the determinants of personal versus impersonal usages are not clear to me. For example, "the" liver, lungs, ovaries, "my" heart, penis, fingers, are commonly heard.

I am not trying to demonstrate that all uses of "the" are distancing or that all uses of "my" mean closeness. Rather, I wish to point out that these words are available to the symbol-using mind when painful material needs handling. When you consistently hear the-the-the-the, the patient is distancing himself or herself from a subject that is painful.

Another example:

All right. Tell me the story of this illness, if you would, please.

Well, it started, a few weeks ago. I was visiting my sister in Rochester. Ah, I wasn't at home. But before I left, I think the very same— the very next day— ah, still there, I was just sitting at the table and suddenly I got a very bad pain in the back of the left leg, about over here. As if, um, maybe a muscle were pulled or something like that— just ached. A Charlie horse—And then that developed so that within two days I could barely stand on that leg. I didn't know whether— I figured it was a muscle—I thought for a moment maybe it's something vascular, but my other leg is the bad leg from the vascular point of view. I had thrombophlebitis in it—this— that's my good leg.

This patient's ability to distance herself from her legs by her use of language is impressive.

Then there is "they." Rather than referring to "my doctor," the patient can shift to the amorphous "they." Further away still are "people," or "doctors," or "those doctors." A patient whose reference to his or her previous hospitalization is always in "they" terms is probably discussing an uncomfortable experience with physicians.

"He" and "she" are employed to avoid speaking about oneself, when the patient says "this boy I know, he ...," but the reference is often really to the speaker. The two articles "the" and "a" also enable gradations of distance. "The" is usually used for something very specific, when the object being discussed has already been mentioned. Shifting to "a" shifts to vagueness: "What does one do to remove a cyst from an ovary," instead of "the cyst from my ovary."

What is the point of physicians knowing about these distancing phenomena? There are three.

The first is that hearing a patient continually use distancing mechanisms tells you that the person, object, disease, or symptom being referred to is a source of pain or fear to the patient. This is the language of denial or avoidance.

Incidentally, such usages are so common that I have begun to believe that denial is the automatic mechanism and nondenial the active process. A patient denying his or her condition may not act on information, take medication, have necessary tests, or surgery. In other words, when denial is present, it seems reasonable to assume that noncompliance will be common. Thus the physician hearing this language is alerted to the possibility of noncompliance. For example, a patient came to see me who had widespread metastatic disease from carcinoma of the breast. She was angry with her previous doctor because, she said, "He would not deal directly with me about my condition." As we discussed her disease, previous therapy, and symptoms, it was apparent that she had placed virtually her entire body off in the distant land of impersonal pronouns: "a," "other," "the." After a while I said, "You are being unfair to your doctor when you accuse him of not being direct and depersonalizing your case, since that is what you have done to yourself." I pointed out her usages and told her that unless she took some of herself and the healthy function of her body back into the space called "I," it was going to be difficult for me to help her.

My second point is that you must make an effort to avoid the usages that seem to distance you from the patient or the disease when that is not your wish. When a patient with an unpleasant disease or prognosis asks questions about himself or herself, the patient is being told something you may not consciously mean to convey when you say, "Well, patients like that," or "Patients like these," or "With a condition like that", instead of, "Patients like you," or "You can be treated as we treat your disease in others," or "Multiple sclerosis is treated by." Once again, as an attentive listener you must also listen to yourself speaking, to make sure that your language usage reflects what you consciously wish to convey.

The third very practical reason for knowing how these distancing phenomena function is that you can use the same mechanisms to accomplish in the listener just what they do for a speaker.

The next example is taken from a discussion between myself and a patient with metastatic disease to the liver from the colon. She knows her diagnosis and is aware, in specific terms, that she has not long to live.

I want to know exactly where do I stand with this? When can I be up and walking around and go home—

That depends on what happens now. You're— you're obviously, now, gettin' better, gettin' stronger.

I see.

Um, a lot of it depends on how you feel about it. A little stronger, then good, fine. 'Cause while I cannot make that liver better, I cannot make that liver better, here or at home, I can keep you in control of your situation, so—

Can you control the liver by medication?

Yah, No— just listen to me. Listen to me carefully, All right, I cannot make that liver get better, I can't keep it from getting worse. I can only keep YOU on top of things, for as long as that liver holds out for you.

Here, I did for her what language allows a person to do for themselves. I took the diseased liver and put it "over there" apart from her: "that liver," "it," "the" (as distinct from "keep *you* in control," "*you're* getting better," "keep *you* on top of things").

I can tell Irwin that the lump on his abdominal wall is "Just a lump, it is not you, it's just a lump," and within limits, it is effective. A patient and I were talking, and she said, "I keep hearing this clicking when I breathe, up in the back of my chest." She knew she had metastatic cancer from the breast and was aware and felt in control of her situation. I said, "That's a fractured rib from some cancer, pay no attention to it. It won't do anything to you," and we went on talking about another subject.

This is an effective tool, useful if you honor its limits. It is simply another aspect of human nature, like the heart or the immune system, which you use to help make people better. Do not expect, however, simply to say some words, and let it go at that. The implication is that you will do your best to maintain the patient as functional and symptom free as possible *despite* the effects of disease. That is part of the deal in the doctor-patient relationship that makes it possible for your words to be effective.

With this last patient my therapeutic goal was that she die well: in control of herself; free of pain, and as free of other symptoms as possible; remaining the person she was, despite her impending death; able to leave her family with goodbye's said and without leaving too much unresolved family business. For a patient to do all those things requires concentrated emotional effort; effort that must not be displaced by fear of suffering or concentration on physical problems that cannot be solved, like the liver, jaundice, or edema. Such concerns must be thrown overboard, cast to the periphery, to enable the patient to keep on top of her situation. To die well, the patient must be distanced from the disease, or that disease will destroy her *self* and not only her body. But she *is* going to die anyway, you may think. True. The difference is between being killed and dying, between being the subject of her disease or the master of her fate. How can I believe she can ever be the master of her fate when the name of fate for her is carcinoma of the colon? That is her fate only in so far as you and I are concerned or in terms of "objective" reality. But in her world, in her subjective world, the world of language, she is master if she can say, "I am."

She did, indeed, die well. She had remarkably little postoperative pain. Almost no medication was required when she was at home. She accomplished what she set out to do: the family was righted again after the stress of her illness and hospitalization, and her husband, who had a history of psychosis, was successfully told what was happening, a difficult and painful matter. With these problems resolved, to the extent possible for her, she started to become weaker. She was admitted to the hospital and was dead within twelve hours. The patient was emotionally functional and competent until the last twenty-four to thirty-six hours. Not a bad death.

The ultimate fate cannot be changed. Everyone dies. As physicians we do the best we can with objective reality, but this is not enough. Given an ominous reality, we can still work in the world of language, in the world of subjectivity, and we can be remarkably effective even after our technical intervention fails.

3

The Logic of Conversation

This chapter has one basic point to make: all normal conversation is logical. With this understanding you will be able to hear not only what people say but also what they really believe. You will begin to hear a person's inner self talk, or even multiple selves in a single speaker; just as we can be of "two minds" about something, we can also follow different trains of thought, each with a compelling logic, simultaneously.

What Is "Logic?"

In this chapter the word "logic" is used to mean a system that relates premises to a conclusion—a way of connecting a series of ideas in order to arrive at another idea. The philosophical field of logic deals with the complexities that can be introduced into systems that relate premises and conclusions. However, while the logic in a conversation can become quite tangled, a simplified general picture of the logic of conversation will be adequate for our purpose.

The point about the logic of conversation is especially important, because many people believe that conversation is illogical or that the mind itself is not logical. If this were really true, no communication could take place. No listener would be able to figure out what one sentence or phrase in a conversation had to do with another. There must be good reasons for such beliefs, and the next example offers one such reason:

Yes Ma'am. What can I do for you?

Uh, I want to try and sort— I think I have to— I am separated from my husband and have been for about three years and I've got four kids to raise, three—three are now at Chaffe School. Adrienne Clausen likes you, um, and recommended you. I haven't been to an internist or a general practitioner in I can't remember how many years. When the kids are sick, I go and see Ted Kolmer. When we have emergencies, we go to various specialists. Uh, I think I have to go into therapy. Um, probably.... I have mixed feelings about it. Um, but I'd like to sort out, if I possibly can, um, how much of it is physical. Um, I checked with my mother, for instance, you know, the kid— I'm forty-five. Um, my mother has had—gone through a ne— nervous breakdown in her thirties. My father was in on Wall Street and there was—you know, etcetera, etcetera.

Mm-hm

Um, I'm an only child, um.... my father died when I was twelve, um.. But, I— I checked with her about, uh, what, when and how she went through menopause. I've been— I've been through, you know. I got— I got my check-ups. I think the last time I went was about four months ago. I thought they routinely took an estrogen level thing. Um, I had regular periods, every four weeks. Um, but I've been going for the las— since late last spring. I lost fifty pounds last spring; I've got another twenty-five to go. Something changed in my metabolism though. Uh, I'm not able to absolutely control my eating; I find that I can't drink very much. Um, I have tried Valium but I'm going hot and cold all the time.

We have met this woman before. In that instance, her conversation was used as an example of a nervous, anxious sounding patient. It was pointed out that she sounded anxious because of her rapid-fire speech rate and high-pitched voice. When the rate was artificially slowed on the tape recorder, the quality of the pausing—short phrases in relation to the pause length—suggested to me that she might also be depressed. Now, when we note the content of her conversation, she does not seem to make much sense: she sounds illogical.

The next example is another patient, whose reasons for the way she takes her medication for hypertension are, to be charitable, unclear:

All righty. Are you taking your medicine?
Nope.
No? Why not?
Eh, that's a long story.
Well, tell me that long st— I'm interested—
No ... All right—
in that long story.
First of all, when I got the prescription, I recognized these pills as thoses little things that I had took years ago from my other doctor, and they didn't work. I thought, "Well, maybe now. My system's changed, maybe they'll work this time." So I tried them. They didn't.

Well, what do you mean it didn't?

I get, uh, very depressed and, uh, I wake up at night and my head is a real roaring mass—sounds like a boiler factory, the noise is terrific.

Well, that pill wasn't for your boiler factory, that pill was for your blood pressure.

Well, I don't know it—but this is the— the fa—

You mean the pill had that effect on you?

Yes, I wake up with a sweat. I didn't drop them altogether, but I took one like every other day, and I finished the prescription, and then I—

Now, when you took it every other day, did it give you that trouble at night?

It still, uh...Well, I felt I should take something to control my pressure, so once in a while I'll have a guilt feeling and take a pill. And then I took a couple from my husband's bottle, you know, he had the same. So, he was taking the medicine, I was taking the medicine, my son was taking the same medicine— I've had—

What's he taking the same medicine for?

For pressure—and I figured, well, one of us, we're gonna start looking for, uh, weapons—uh, who's gonna take the gun, who's gonna take the knife—

Well, you're all having the—

We're all upset—

—reaction to it?

—So, I stopped taking them, and then my husband called, you said he could stop, and then my son stopped them.

Now nobody's taking them

Mm—

How's everybody's blood pressure, huh?

(Laughing) I don't know; I don't take it. . . . (Sigh)

What is heavens name is she talking about: "Who's gonna get the gun, whose gonna get the knife . . ."? This is the kind of conversation that makes physicians say that nothing "straight" can be obtained from patients, that patients make no sense, do not tell the truth, and produce conversation of little clinical relevance. Consequently many physicians believe that there is little of value to be obtained from talking with patients or from taking a detailed history.

It is odd but true that for the complaint that patients make no sense to be valid, patients must, in some way, be different from the rest of us. Otherwise, we would be saying that we do not make sense either, and most people get quite annoyed when you suggest that they are speaking nonsense.

I have been saying, however, that all conversation has a logic; that conversation is characterized by premises related to each other and to conclusions. The previous two examples do not seem to support my contention, so let me present an intermediate case: a conversation that does not seem logical but which makes absolute sense.

I have been taking Dalmane at your recommendation and being fearful of taking it too much or becoming addicted to it—not knowing anything about drugs and never before taking even aspirin unless I absolutely had to, I take a good portion of it out.
You empty the capsule out!
Correct.
Why don't you just take a blank capsule?
Well, . . . So I'm stupid.

If she had said "I have been taking Dalmane at your suggestion and I empty a good portion of it out," we might wonder why she bothered to take it in the first place. We might speculate endlessly in order to explain her action, which otherwise seems odd. In this instance, speculation is unnecessary because the patient not only gives us her conclusion, "I empty a good portion of it out," but, in the embedded clause, she also provides some of the premises that lead to her conclusion: (1) you recommended Dalmane, but (2) I am fearful of taking too much, and (3) I am fearful of becoming addicted, and (4) I have no knowledge about drugs that might counteract those fears ("not knowing anything about drugs"), such that (5) I have never even taken aspirin unless I absolutely had to, therefore (6) "I take a good portion of it out."

The doctor exaggerates her response by saying "Why didn't you just take a blank capsule?" But this is not what she said. In fact there are still some premises missing, to explain why she took any of the medication at all. We might speculate that she was having trouble sleeping, or that she respected the physician and thus, despite her fears, tried taking the Dalmane. While we cannot know those things with certainty, the example makes clear that an utterance which may, at first, seem odd, may be logical nonetheless. The utterance is logical, because it contains a cohesive set of premises compatible with the stated conclusion.

This next example also seems odd at first:

Will aspirin sometimes relieve them?
Uh, never completely, but it helps a little sometimes . . . . I sort of don't like to take it, it's sort of a . . .

Why?
(Pause) Even when it helps a little, I know the headache's still there . . . It's sort of—the pain's been deadened.

Most of us who take aspirin for a headache do so in the hope that the pain will be deadened. But this patient does not like aspirin for this very reason! This does not make sense; it does not seem logical. Some people, however, are not satisfied with merely symptom relief, and say, "Don't just take away symptoms, try to get at the cause." If this patient had said, "The pain's been deadened, but I know the cause must still be there, and that's what I want to get at," we might disagree, but his remark would make perfect sense. Again, in the next example a patient makes the kind of statement that is commonly labeled illogical:

The only reason why I cut out the dairy products is because I was allergic to penicillin.
Yeah. But penicillin doesn't have anything to do with it. But, you know, there are some times when—
Yeah, but penicillin is made from dairy products.
Wha—who who told you? Who told you that? Who told you that one?
Isn't it?
No!

The patient provides a perfectly sensible reason for not taking dairy products when one is allergic to penicillin: "penicillin is made from dairy products." He is not lacking in logic, he is merely incorrect. These last two examples of the sort of utterances that are often taken to be "nonsense" are not without logical coherence. They have premises that lead systematically to a conclusion. Some of their premises are wrong, however.

This is the first reason that everyone does not realize that all normal conversation is logical: errors in information are mistaken for errors in logic. If one or all of the premises are incorrect in a logical system, the conclusion will usually be wrong, no matter how faultless the logic. And when the conclusion is wrong, it sounds "dumb," "silly," "nonsensical." The hearer could just as easily be the one with incorrect information, yet might believe the speaker to be "illogical."

As these patients speak, they tell us something about their beliefs; they convey ideas and information that help us care for them. These ideas and information are contained in the premises of their respective utterances, although they are not "the point" of their comments.

One man's remark suggested that he believed in getting at the causes of things, he thought this more important than merely deadening headache pain. In treating him, you would have to address this belief, because if he thought his medication was simply for symptomatic relief, he might not take it. He might not take his steroids if he had asthma, because his belief about causes might be very different from the physician's. The patient gave the doctor such information as part of an utterance about aspirin. Another patient provided information about her fear of medication and addiction. Just as hearers tend not to hear the specific words employed by a speaker or to be aware of the paralanguage of someone's speech, so too hearers tend to lose a speaker's premises, leaving only the conclusion hanging in the air. More is lost than simply the unheard premise. Premises exist as parts of a system of beliefs about the world, and the belief system of a person tells a great deal about that person.

Uncovering "Hidden" Premises and Conclusions

Let us examine another facet of the problems that arise when a listener does not separate observation (what the listener hears) from interpretation (what the listener thinks the speaker means).

Sometimes a speaker will present a conclusion that appears incorrect and then will gradually provide the premises that support the conclusion. In this next example, the patient's wife asked me for a prescription for "American lithium" for her husband. Why American? lithium is lithium, is it not? No, not for this patient.

... said to me. And he said, "Look, we— Eric Cassell's going to fix up Fernando's lithium. Because the lithium in our— in our country, we don't know if it's as good as the lithium which you have here. Perhaps for this—

This meaning—?

Ups and downs. You see, this is our lithium. That's what he takes—

How long has he been on lithium, nine months now?

Eh, yes, since November, no?

All right. Well the— th—the first question is . . . . . . lithium is lithium.

Mm. Eh, yes.

It's a simple drug. It's a simple salt. It is not a sophisticated drug.

Mm.

There should be no problem—I mean, I could write a prescription for lithium and—it's

Yes.

American lithium . . . but, uh, in all honesty, I think it should be no different.
No?

Okay. So the first question is—which is raised is: Is—is there a possibility that your lithium and our lithium are different?
That is it.

And we think a very small possibility.
Small.

Very small. So that's the first question. It actually is, you know, nowadays, uh, the same drugs are all over the world.
All over the world, huh?

And that's good!
But, what we have is the, not the— the serious, eh, chemical men who do the—the pills. And, I know my father had, eh, gout . . . and he

Mm-hm.
came over to Boston and they gave him— they told him, "You have to have this . . . Colchicine" . . . in those days.

Mm-hm.
And he had Colchicine in Buenos Aires and the gout was the same. And he ga— came from North America the— the medicine— It was better. And we gave to

It was better?
our man in the camp, and he was . . . enchanted with that medicine and with the other one, it didn't work. So, that's why we're . . . And the lithium?

Now we come to the lithium.
Right.

Which brand lithium will you use? Now, there is a difference in purity there— that could be—
That can be, now, you see. I'm sure it can be.

Oh, yes.

Once the premises were teased out, the meaning of "American lithium" becomes clear: A drug that has been carefully manufactured and quality controlled.

There are more interesting and sophisticated reasons why we do not hear a speaker's logic. For example, the premise is stated but not heard.

Any shortness of breath?
No, uh, just once, uh, you know, I got so busy, I forgot to take those water pills for two mornings.

And, what happened then?

And, it was very humid out and I . . . I was not short of breath but, you know, I wasn't breathing—

You knew there was a difference?

I knew there was a difference, shall I say, because, uh, normally my breathing doesn't bother me—I'm not conscious of it.

Mm-hm.

And, uh, Friday—I have a pill case, you know, I take so many for the week—two of them a day—But I had six pills left. On Friday.

And you—

And I realized what I'd forgotten to do.

Why was this woman short of breath? Most listeners believe it is because she did not take her diuretic. Without the diuretic she reaccumulated some fluid, went back into congestive heart failure, and was, consequently, short of breath. But she did not discover she had failed to take her medication until Friday, when she noticed that she had six pills left in the pill case. To what did she attribute her dyspnea earlier in the week? Try this on some listeners, and you will find that they are slow to come to "the humidity" as the reason. Once you accept the fact that conversation is logical, it follows that premises are never thrown into the utterance unless they serve the underlying logic. In this case we have to explain what the phrase, "it was very humid out," is doing in the sentence that describes her dyspnea. She must have related the humidity to her difficulty in breathing. The remainder of her utterance makes the point explicitly.

Well, it's almost like a good test, isn't it?

Yes, it really was.

Mm-hu

Because I was laying it down to the humidity and all, you know.

Thus, when a speaker says A, and B, and C, and X, and D, and therefore E, the premise that seems so much out of place is often forgotten by listeners: they simply do not hear it. After all, what has X got to do with it? The misplaced premise, X, may make no sense to the listener (and then be forgotten), but it is important to the logical stream of the speaker, or it would not be included in the utterance. Just as words do not appear in conversation randomly, neither do premises. As your skill as a listener increases, so too will your ability to hear every premise and follow the flow of the speakers logic.

Like the verb in a German sentence, the premise sometimes appears at the end of the utterance. Until it appears, nothing may make much sense. In the next example, the fact that the dialogue is quite long helps make my point.

The problem really is this: um, I've been to two different endocrinologists, and in both cases nobody'll TELL me anything! And, um—
What do you mean they won't tell you anything.
They won't tell me anything. It's like—
They must tell you SOMEthing. They must—
—you, know, they go, "mmmmmm" or "Hmmmmm—" . . .
Do they—
I-it-it's like you always get the feeling that you're sort of getting the bum's rush out of the office, and you never know the difference. And wha-what I'm concerned about is this:—I'm a flutist, right?
Mm-hm.
And a lot of what you do in music is sort of bound up with things like reflexes. And—
Mm-hm,
I notice, for instance, when I start slowing down, now— now I'm doing a job which is the Goldman Band. We sight-read half of each concert we play.—Which means I don't see the music I'm going to play until I'm actually performing it.
Mm-hm.
And that's a kind of complex eye-to-hand— In other words . . .
You're one beat behind the—
Yo—
—rest of the orchestra?
Well, (laughing) it's almost that bad! But, you know, it's just—
So you go to these guys and what do they actually tell you?
Very little. (Laughs)
Well, they must tell you something, Bettie . . .
Well, you know, I-I get upset because— The last doctor I went to is a very nice lady, and I'm sure very competent. But I always get the feeling, I m-m-maybe it is I-I-yi-I get intimidated and I don't feel like I can say, "Would you please take time and TELL me . . ." you know.
Well, did she tell—
Ah-m—
—you to raise your dose or lower it?
Well, what I— What I've been taking is two-and-a-half of Synthroid.
Mm-hm

—Yellow Synthroid.

How long had that been?

Uhh.... about ... about a year-and-a-half. We were doing two and then about, I guess, six months ago, she upped it to two-and-a-half.

Mm-hm

Um, the other thing—

You only use—I see.

—is that my periods have been totally irregular. You know, th-they never have straightened out. She said, "Let's wait six months," and we waited over six months and—they've been everything from twenty-four days to thirty-nine days and never the same thing two months in a row.

Mm-hm

The end result of which is that, you know, my hair and my skin have been super oily and— and, you know, that I expect. But, it just, you know, it's like . . . you know, for one week it's clear and the next week it's all broken out and oily and, you know, just—

Does that happen at the same time as your reflexes slowing down?

I haven't really been able to correlate that much. I guess what I'm saying is, I know there are a certain number of ups and downs in my body, but is this trip really necessary? I feel like I'm getting—

Which trip are we—

—too many ups and downs.

Talking about, the trip of your reflexes or the trip of yor skin—?

Both of them, both of them.

If I—If your—

Because they've been a constant problem.

—reflexes came back to normal, but your skin stayed the way it was—

Mm-mm.

—would you be only half satisfied?

I suppose I could live with it if I have to.

If your skin came back to normal but your—

(beginning to laugh)

—reflexes stayed—

(Laughing)

Huh?

You mean, I've gotta have it—a fast choice, huh? I can't have it both ways . . . (laughing)

You don't have that fast choice. I'm trying to find out what the problem is. You see, I know that if the problem was—

There are two problems, essentially.
—solely—If the problem was solely—
Mm-hm,
uh— "Am I on the right dose of thyroid?"
Yeah
—and both of those endocrinologists are perfectly capable of telling you to raise or lower your dose . . .
Mm-hm,
—since somehow or other that has not been an adequate answer, then maybe they didn't hear the question.
Ja.
So I wanna make sure I hear the questions.
Okay. There are really two things going on. I'm saying essentially, the one that's the very most important to me is the thing that affects my livelihood, you know.
Mm-hm.
I don't like the feeling of walking into a rehearsal and not being able to concentrate, not being able to think, feeling slow, feeling my reflexes slow down. My tongue slows down. Everything.
Mm-hm.
It's all coordination in music. All of it. And, I don't like that. What I'm also saying is that I want to get myself into some kind of opti— con— you know, as— as good a physical condition as I can because I may be auditioning for the New York Philharmonic next year, and I'd like to be put together—
Right!
—if you don't, you know—If you don't mind, please! (Laughs)

What neither doctor had heard in her previous visits was the last sentence. The premise underlying this endless conversation had to do with auditioning for the New York Philharmonic. She was concerned, understandably, that she do her best, and she wondered whether the apparent slowing of her musical reflexes was related to her thyroid function. You may feel that sitting through that long dissertation would be impossible for the busy practitioner, a true waste of time. But two endocrinologists really did waste their time, because they did not hear her out. Two wasted visits. Wasted money, doctors' time, and patient's time. At the very least inefficient listening is not cost-effective.

One cannot be sure that the patient mentioned her concerns about the Philharmonic to the endocrinologists. Making a doctor's visit, however, is in itself a statement of a conclusion: "I need to go to the doctor." When the reasons for the visit are not clear, they must be elicited. Adjusting her dose of Synthroid could have been done over the telephone, if the problem were that simple. Moreover the early part of the conversation, in which she says "I've been to two endocrinologists, and nobody'll tell me anything," suggests that she did raise her concerns, at least to some degree, but that they were not addressed by the physicians. Further, while I say that the basic point is not explicitly made until the very end, she introduces her worries about her musical abilities and reflexes within the first few exchanges: "What I'm concerned about is this: I'm a flutist, right?" and then she tells of her difficulties. What is not obvious, and becomes even less so when she talks about her skin, is what the basic problem is: the Philharmonic audition. A more alert physician might have asked in the beginning of the interaction, "Why are your musical reflexes a matter of concern now?" The audition would probably have surfaced earlier, the problem could have been discussed in her terms, and the visit have ended sooner, with a satisfied patient.

It seems more than reasonable to ask why the patient did not directly tell the endocrinologist what was bothering her. She could have said, "I am going to have a Philharmonic audition next year, and I am afraid that my slowed reflexes will hurt my chances. Do you think it is my thyroid?" However, she may not have known what really bothered her, for many reasons. The problem may relate to an unconscious conflict, so that the reason is inaccessible to her awareness. It may mean something so important that, by avoiding the words, she protects herself from fears and concerns that would be difficult to handle. She may be intimidated by doctors and become inarticulate in their presence. Physical illness may be very frightening to her. You can probably think of many more reasons, from conscious to unconscious and back again. Patients do not always know or tell the doctor why they have come, yet if the doctor is to get the job done, the patients' concerns and fears must be uncovered. One of the best ways of knowing what is troubling a patient, when it is not otherwise obvious, is to follow the logic of a conversation.

This example brings up another point. A delayed premise is almost always heralded by repetitious speech. The patient went over the same ground repeatedly. Whenever a person talks over and over about the same thing, then the important premise has probably not yet been stated. You will have to either elicit or wait for it. Here is another example of repetitious speech that occurs because the important premise does not surface until late:

Everything is healed up nicely. Uh, it's not unusual to have this kind of . . . continuous abnormal bleeding when you're breast feeding because your ovary is suppressed. It's not working while you're breast feeding for at least—for many, many months. So you don't have the proper hormonal stimulation to the womb so you have this kind of staining. I can treat it with some pills but I don't like to do that while you're breast feeding because sometimes medication comes out—

In the milk?

In the milk, do you see?

Mm-hm.

I would wait a little while longer, okay? Before your— before we treat it with any medication. If it doesn't clear up spontaneously in a few more weeks, you can call me on the phone, and I'll give you some pills to take for five days that will tend to get rid of this abnormal bleeding.

I can't take this while I'm nursing, c-could I?

Well, you can. The only problem is they say sometimes some of it does come out in the, uh—

I will not take the chance.

—in the milk. It doesn't pay to take a chance because it's not a serious, uh, problem, at least for a couple of more weeks. I'd wait a few more weeks before I would do anything. Then if it doesn't clear up, let's say, in two weeks, call me on the phone—you don't have to come in—and I'll order some pills for you to take for five days which will clear out any of this tissue that's built up from the breast feeding and then you'll be nice and clean.

Uh, that will be even while I'm breast feeding?

Yeah. Yeah.

What would that—what will happen then if I'm— you know, . . . because—

No. What I mean is this; if we have to do it, we'll do it. We'll wait a few more weeks. We can't let you just keep bleeding continuously forever.

R-right.

In a few more weeks, if it hasn't stopped by itself, we'll take the little bit of a risk involved, and just give you five pills.

What kind of risk is that? I mean, what is this—

Practically zero.

You know, for us there is a risk. I mean, no one likes to take any kind of—I'd rather stop breast feeding than take any kind of risk.

Oh, I don't think the risk is that high that you need to be concerned about it. It's only for five days, you see, that you'll be taking the pills. In fact, we could probably squeeze them in in three days.

So what if I wouldn't nurse for three days. I just, let's say, uh—

Well I don't think it'll make that much difference. At this dosage the small amount that'll come—even if some comes through, it should have no ill effect on the baby anyway.

But there's a chance, you're sure you want me to take it, a small chance—

That's up to you to decide but, uh, I certainly wouldn't give you any medication at least for a few more weeks since it's only eight weeks.

Mm-hm.

And many, many people do this at eight weeks. So I would wait at least another two weeks before even considering any kind of treatment.

Okay. What kind of medication. That's the Provera?

Exactly.

Mm-hm. Well, because you gave it to me last time, too.

Yes, you can take like two a day for three days instead of one a day for five days—

For five days.

—you see, like that. Okay?

Okay, so you want to wait another two weeks then.

Sure.

Okay—

There's no rush, and, uh, th-the— most often this will clear up spontaneously by eight or ten weeks.

Well, this used to happen to me but would be staining, light staining, where this is bleeding, it's—

I think it's simply a hormonal thing—

Yeah?

—and you see this, as I say, in people who are breast feeding.

I must ask you one thing about Provera. Is this— uh, I know what I read in the Times, uh—

No, this is not estrogen—

—a month ago.

No, this has nothing to do with what you read in the Times with the—

I'm just—

—bad results with Estrogen. Premarin is what you're thinking of.

I don't know, I just read something so I'm trying, you know, I wanna ask you before I, uh—

No, that's the uh— that's Premarin. That's another hormone.

Okay. Fine. For that, I trust you, and I hope you're not—don't laugh. I just, you know, if you don't know something like—

That's right.

—find out.

It's good to ask.

The woman seems unable to accept reassurance. First, the physician does not want to give her medication to suppress the postpartum vaginal staining. Then, when she does not want the prescription, he attempts to reassure her of its safety. Not a chance. Around and around the conversation goes, without coming to closure. She asks the question, he answers the question, but back comes the same question again. Whenever this happens, I believe it is because the true question has not yet been answered (or, perhaps, even asked). Here, the matter at issue seems to be the appearance of the medication in breast milk, but I think that is not what bothers her. It turns out that she is quite familiar with Provera, having taken it many times before. Indeed, what seems to be worrying her is whether Provera is the hormone she read about in the *New York Times* that causes cancer. When the obstetrician talks directly to this fear, making it clear that Provera is not an estrogen, she is finally reassured and the conversation can end. After all, she had taken Provera many times before and may well have worried that she was already at increased risk for cancer.

Perhaps the conversation ended, because she became weary of asking the same question over and over again and finally settled for his last answer. Patients usually do not indicate true closure unless they mean it. If you wonder about this, ask patients whether you have answered the question that bothered them. "Do you have any other questions?" or "Is there anything else bothering you, that you would like me to answer?" I think physicians are often afraid of asking such questions, because of the time that may be consumed if they ever give the patient the chance to ask questions or because of the possibility that the patient will ask questions they cannot answer. Both are realistic fears, but such situations occur infrequently and can be handled. Much more frequently, the patient will feel that the doctor has been concerned, understanding, and open. And in many cases the patient's needs will be more fully met. This seems well worth the extra time required, especially since in the long run time is more often saved than wasted when patients' questions are answered.

In this next example the underlying premise never surfaces. What do you think was neither asked nor answered?

Hello. What can I do for you?
Well, I hope you could do something. Um, I had a plantar wart removed—what possessed me to do it, I don't know—uh, but anyway, last December, and it just—has—been—no—END of problem! It, uh— I mean, do you want me to go into all the details?
Well, w-ju-well just tell me what's bothering you about it now.
It hurts.

Mm-hm.

And it keeps opening up. I mean, it heals, uh, I think it's going to heal, and then it just looks like, well, not a scab, but, uh, you know, the skin, like the skin looks different, like there's a whitish area around it and then it'll open again and it hurts. And it's been just doing this on and off for—

Well, let me just—

—a long, like, you know, quite a while.

—let me take a look at it.... This was um, when, in December.

December.

Uh, in the office.

Mm...And it's sort of gone through various stages of, uh, development.

Have you been, um, wearing anything on it? Uh, you know, like, like a dressing on it...?

No, I haven't been wearing anything on it lately. Except for a Band aid because, you know, the stocking— you, it does secrete something and, and the stocking sticks to it.

Mm.

It just doesn't seem to want to heal and it's most...upsetting.

Mm-hm. Yeah. Well...you see, the problem is, well, you see, there's probably still some of the plantar wart in there. Uh, and I would think, it certainly feels like it. Secondly, if it's not going to heal very well. Well, you know, walking on it, and so forth, keeps pressure on...keeps opening up...Uh...

You mean, it's never going to heal?

Oh, well,...Uh, I suppose eventually it would but...I think there are a few things we might do to try to help it, but, I mean, I don't think there— there's anything about it that—don't do anything about the plantar wart remaining.

Just f-forget it?

Well, I think the thing at the moment is, you know, that would help it most is, uh, if you put a little, if you put a little donut over it. That would, that—

Mm-hm.

—would sort of...put your weight on it right here, you see, and it'll leave the area where, well, where the drainage comes out, where— where it's open, so that it's, it's free of any pressure when you walk. I th— I kn— I kn— I think that would be the thing to, well, to try for a while, try t— try to take the pressure off and see if it won't heal, uh, spontaneously, 'cause, uh—I mean, it looks clean even though it drains a little bit. I— an— and, it looks clean. I— it should heal, you know, if it's given the opportunity to. It's I guess just—I mean, being on it keeps it, keeps it from healing, and since there, there is some plantar wart in there, uh it tends not to heal as if there weren't any in there, so, maybe we can put a little donut on it, a-and why don't we see how that goes for a while.

And then, uh ... it— it'll just, uh, I mean it will, w— y-you know, I don't quite understand. In other words, you think that just eventually time would heal it? Is that what you're saying? 'Cause after all, it's been after all a very long time.

Well, I'm n— there are certain things that—

I mean, it doesn't make any difference whether I bathe it or I put anything on it, or— or the whole thing doesn't make any difference?

Well, you see, it-i-it's basically not very healthy tissue— not that it's infected or anything, but it's— it's— it's plantar wart tissue. Uh, it doesn't—

(Sigh)

—tend to heal as rapidly as, say, well,—I mean if you cut your hand or, or—or it's som— or you broke your, you know, like that.

Uh-hn. I— I hate to say, I think you're the ninth doc— I can never go to doctors, you know, unless I'm dragged in, and you're the eighth or ninth. I could write up catalogs just—

But I wouldn't do

I don't know.

—do anything more with it. Just, uh, just protect it.

And, uh, you have no idea how long it will take to heal?

Oh. That's really hard to say. Uh, uh, sometimes they heal very rapidly, you know, and all of a sudden— They'll be indolent for months on end, and then in a two week period they'll heal up. Uh, sometimes they drag on for several months. I think if you (sigh) protect it, uh, it won't do too badly. Uh, but don't, um—

But, you're not, you're not telling me I'm going to have to go through life with this, I mean, with a problem with my foot.

Oh, no—

No?

—No, no, no. I would think, I mean, I would think it would heal up if you pro— protected it like that. I mean, the less you meddle with it, clearly the better off you are.

Just . . . leave it . . . alone.

Okay?

Well, I'm . . .

but it's not serious.

No. No. W-well why don't you let me take a look at it in a month or so, and you can make an appointment with my secretary.

I think she was afraid the wound that would not heal was cancer. How would you have dealt with her? Why not say: "This is not cancer. It is a plantar wart. It may look awful, it may take weeks to heal, but it is not cancer. I know that one of the seven danger signs of cancer is an unhealing wound, but some wounds don't heal because they have plantar wart tissue in them, not because of cancer. Period! Put a donut on it to take the pressure off, leave it alone, and give it more time." If this were not the patient's worry, she could always say so. This was one of the longest interactions we recorded in that particular surgeon's office. He saw thirteen patients in fifty-four minutes and dealt with their problems warmly and efficiently. This patient, however, took longer than patients with carcinoma of the breast, gall bladder disease, or duodenal ulcer. The point is, when a patient cannot be reassured, the problem that is of concern has not been addressed. When we deal with speech that is vague in its reference, we will discover another reason why this surgeon's speech was not very reassuring.

Just as premises may be unspoken, conclusions, too, may be unvoiced. Consider the following:

It may be a little high.
Is it a little high?
Yeah, you seem to be a little tense.
Huh?
You seem to be nervous. Are you?
Yeah—
Is there anything bothering you?
Well, there has been—I try not to let anything worry— but, my husband died because he was a worry wart and I said now I'll never die of a heart attack. But, uh, the thing is now, see, my son, he has a place down in Breezy Point and he took the family and his wife—
Breezy Point is which way? The Rockaways?
That's Rock— yeah.
Yeah—
And I'm all alone in the house—not that I'm afraid, but the thing is you hear so many sudden deaths—you know what I mean? And I'm all alone. And I fell—gee, I could—and I have to watch my step, too. I mi— I fall easily if I'm not—don't wat— don't watch my step. So I don't, uh—
Yeah.
—seem to, uh ... I'm a little upset and, uh, 'cause every once in a while I get a pain up in my ... up here, you know—
Mm-hm.
But, uh, I try not to worry about anything. I say whatever comes, comes.
Well, I mean, uh ...
Did it go up much, the blood pressure?
No.
Yeah.

Not much . . . Well, you have to find a way—
But I seem—I'm shi— I seem tense to you, don't I?
Yes.
But I think it might be this. I was a little hurt—
Mm.
—at my son. 'Cause he didn't tell me where he was going—
Uh-huh.
—with his family.
Uh-huh.
I have an idea he had shared it with the dau— my daughter-in-law
has some sisters out on the Island, out in Bay— Hampton Bays and
that. But what harm would it have been? I thought he was going to
call me up before he left yesterday morning, and he didn't.
I wouldn't, uh— in your place, I wouldn't be that meticulous.
No.
—Too grown up for this . . . Right? Don't let those little things—
But-but-but what harm would it be—
—get on your nerves.
—He says, well, eh, "And I'll be home at such-and-such a time" or
something like that over the weekend. I don't know how long they
were going.
Yeah.
And WHERE they were going, you see. That was the only thing that
bothered me.
Mm-hm.
'Cause I has heard f-for the last few weeks I've heard so many people
that dropped dead, you know—
Well, it doesn't mean that—
—and then it annoys me.
There is no such thing as an epidemic of—
—You understand? Panic.
—people dropping dead—
Oh, I know—
—all of a sudden. Dead all of a sudden.
No. But, then, well, of course—
*What happens to other people doesn't necessarily mean it is going to happen to
you, you know.*
To you, no. But, when the weather is nice and clear, I do feel very
good, but when it's like—last week it was 86
Oh, yeah. Well, everybody—

—and 88, that was, uh—

—*was sick last*—

. . . then I just feel like, I don't know what.

Yeah. Well, okay. Uh, keep taking the pills and put the collar . . . and, uh, let's check on those tests.

That's when I'll see. I see.

Yeah. And we'll see how they do.

Her son may have known best, when he did not tell his mother where he was going for the weekend. The conclusion, although never spoken, is perfectly clear. She tells us the whole familiar story: "My son neglects me. My pressure is up. I could die. Nobody would know I died. I'm alone. I'm abandoned. I'm afraid." Inexperienced listeners, hearing this recording, are often impatient with the amount of the doctor's time that this patient is wasting with a problem about which the doctor can do nothing—and besides, this is not his job! Many physicians who have heard this segment (which was recorded in a clinic) are relieved to hear that the same thing goes on in other doctors' offices. But this doctor, in common with most, did not know what to say, so he ended on a medical note: take these pills. He does his best to be comforting and spends considerable time trying to reassure the patient but probably not very effectively. The doctor was not aware that to address directly the underlying question not only ends the conversation efficiently but is also very reassuring. The patient knows that the doctor cannot make her son be more loving or attentive. If he had correctly identified what was troubling her, however, the doctor would have established the fact that he understood her concerns. Once again, I am suggesting that addressing the problem of the inattentive son will shorten, rather than lengthen, the conversation. Do not take this on faith. Instead, try it yourself. It will either work or not, and you will not lose much in the attempt. I believe, although I cannot be sure, that demonstrating understanding in situations like this is reassuring, even when nothing else is done, because a person who is understood by another feels connected to that other. Of this I am sure, however: demonstrating understanding may enable the physician to obtain an accurate history, when this would otherwise be impossible. On one occasion I was making rounds as a visiting professor when a patient was presented who had been admitted the night before with the diagnosis of orthostatic hypotension. Although some of its manifestations are common, the disease orthostatic hypotension is quite unusual. As the details of the history of this black woman in her forties were presented to me, my doubts about the diagnosis increased. When the family history was finally presented, I learned that the patient's mother had been admitted to another hospital for a heart attack. "How long ago?" I asked the intern. "Three days." "When did the patient's symptoms start?" "Three days ago." To me, the probability that she had orthostatic hypotension plummeted even further. Coincidences like this are very suspicious. "Who is taking care of the family now that the patient's mother is in the hospital?" It turned out that the entire burden had fallen on this patient, since the mother usually cared for the family. The case presentation was taking place in the hallway. (Some physicians like to hear the history at the bedside but I do not: I want to be free to ask questions of those who care for the patient. Further I need time to think before I get to the bedside.) We went into her room, and there was this sad-looking woman sitting on the edge of her bed. My opening line was, "You poor lady. That whole family has fallen right on your shoulders now, and here you've gotten sick. Isn't that..." I did not finish speaking before tears began streaming down her face. There was the case! With a few more questions I was able to establish that her symptoms were the same as her mother's and elicit additional information that put an end to the diagnosis of orthostatic hypotension.

As we left the patient's room, the physician who had invited me to the medical school said, "You certainly were lucky to have the whole case open up right in front of you." Lucky, indeed! I had planned my opening line from the moment I heard about the coincidence between the mother's heart attack and the onset of the patient's symptoms. When I saw the sad look on her face, I went ahead as planned. You can ask a patient from now until Doomsday, "Did you get sick because your mother left the burden on your shoulders?" and you will never find out anything. A person who admitted to this would be admitting a moral fault: the failure to assume responsibility. You should not worry about such moral issues; what you need is the information that will help get them well again. This woman, for example, needed some help with her burdens while her mother was ill before she could be made better and discharged from the hospital. Many would argue that her symptoms were "psychological," and thus not in the realm of the internist. I do not find such distinctions very useful because what I am always trying to discover is what I must do to make patients better, return them to function. The story points up the fact that by demonstrating understanding with the patient's plight, the necessary history was obtained for getting her better again.

What I chose to say as my opening line I learned through experience derived from years of listening to patients' conversations. Who has not heard someone bemoan the burdens heaped on them by outrageous fortune, in this instance the mother's heart attack. Everything that you learn about how the world works and how people live their lives should become part of your "medical" knowledge. I acquired much of this information from taking histories. The process is similar to the way I learned what the abdomen feels like in health and disease.

We have seen that the logic of a conversation—the thread that connects the ideas together—may not be obvious, because the basic premise comes late in the conversation or because the premise is unspoken, or is there, but we do not hear it. Where the premise is unspoken, the failure of the conversation to reach closure—to come to any satisfactory conclusion—signals that the real issue is not being attended to. Further I have suggested that speaking to those hidden premises does not necessarily lengthen, and indeed may shorten, the time required for conversing.

The logical nature of an utterance may be obscured because the listener does not "hear" what the speaker actually said. This is different from not taking into account the reference to humidity by the patient who was short of breath. There the listener remembers the words when reminded. In the present case the listener does not believe that he or she ever heard the words. Every physician knows that patients and families can be told something very clearly and then behave as though they had never heard what was said. This is particularly true when bad news is first broken. Laypersons often deny that anything like this ever occurs. Instead, they blame doctors, who "never tell you anything." For example, in one case, in fact of the patient's denial, his wife could not believe that Fred was unaware of his cancer. After all the things that had been said and that had happened, it would be impossible for him not to know. Yet she then asked, "Doctor, why didn't you tell me that Fred had cancer when the biopsy report came back?" "But Sara, I did tell you, don't you remember?" "Of course you didn't tell me, doctor. It would be impossible for me to forget such a thing!"

The next two examples display the phenomenon in pure form. This patient visited the surgeon's office in the morning and late that afternoon saw the internist. It was a happy accident that both physicians were being recorded on that day. Here is the entire transcript of the visit to the surgeon.

Did you see Dr. Cassell?

Uh, yeah. I hadn't seen him for three weeks. I have to see him tonight. Yes, he's seen this.

All right. Okay.

In fact, I think it looks slightly better than the last time you've seen it.

Have you been keeping any kind of a dressing on it at all?

Yeah, I've been keeping gauze pads on it. And I've been, you know, changing them frequently and putting hot water on it. Before it got so big, I figured that maybe it would just, you know, by cleaning it, and keeping it dry, it would close.

Okay, I think, um, I think probably it would be, uh, desirable to keep it, keep it covered. I think you could put like a little Vaseline on it, though—

Uh-huh.

—rather than just a dry dressing. And then maybe you could let me take a look at it in about a week or so, huh?

Sure.

And I'll talk to Dr. Cassell about it too. Okay—

Okay.

I am not really quite sure what it is, but I— i—i-it looks nice and clean. I think it probably will just heal up by itself given the time.

It's been a couple of months. That's what I was worried about.

Yeah. Well, let's watch it a little while and see. If it doesn't, we can always close it up but, for the moment let's see if it won't do this by itself.

Less than eight hours later when the patient saw me, the following conversation took place. Purely by chance I had listened to the recording of the morning visit.

Mm.

Did Dr. Dineen call you?

Mm-hm. So . . . ?

So, what did he say? To me, he said absolutely nothing.

Nothing?

Nothing . . . "Come back—"

What do you mean, "Nothing?"

"I'll see— I'll see you next week."

He didn't even tell you what he thought would happen?

No.

Or what he wanted to do about it or anything? He—

Not a thing.

—didn't tell you what it was?
Nope.
Well, he said to me, "I think it'll close by itself."
Good!
He said, "If it's necessary, we can close it but, I think it'll close by itself." He didn't tell you that?
Nope.
Mm-hm.
In!—Out!

There it is in black and white! I have always wanted to ask the patient about it, to play the two segments for her and see what she thinks now. But, I have not. Incidentally, the nonhealing wound turned out to be pyoderma gangrenosum, a complication of ulcerative colitis, which occurred even though she had had a total colectomy many years earlier. The wound did not close for three years!

Sorting Mixed Premises

In opening this chapter, an example was used to demonstrate why physicians and others often believe conversation, the mind, or people to be illogical. That person seemed to just pour out words, phrases, sentences as though they were unrelated, giving her speech an illogical, chaotic quality. Let us consider her speech again:

Yes, Ma'am. What can I do for you?
(Sigh) Since late last spring—I lost fifty pounds last spring—I've got another twenty-five to go. Something changed in my metabolism, though. Um, I'm not able to absolutely control my eating; I find that I can't drink very much. Um, but I'm going hot and cold all the time. Um, I checked with my mother. But I— I checked with her about, ah, what, when, and how she went through menopause. Um, I have regular periods, every four weeks. Um, I've been—I've been to, you know— I get, I get my check-ups. I haven't been to an internist or general practitioner in—I can't remember how many years. When the kids are sick, we go and see Ted Kramer. When we have emergencies, we go to various specialists. Um, I think the last time I went was about four months ago. —I thought they routinely took an estrogen level thing. My mother has had—gone through a ne— nervous breakdown in her thirties. You know, I can'— I'm forty-five. Um, I have separated from my husband and have been for about three years—
Mm-hm.

—and I've got four kids to raise, three—three are now at Chaffe School. I'm an only child. Um, my father was in on Wall Street and there was—you know, etcetera, etcetera.

Mm-hm.

My father died when I was twelve. Um ... I have tried Valium. I think I have to go into therapy, um, probably ... and I'm trying— I have mixed feelings about it. Um, but I'd like to sort out, if I POSSIBLY can, um, how much of it is physical.

As you may notice, I switched around the phrases but left nothing out. I put premises that were logically related alongside each other: all those relating to physical health, her metabolism, and the possibility of menopause were included in the early part of the conversation; farther on were included subjects that might relate to her mental health—her mother's nervous breakdown, the stresses of raising four children as a single parent, the early death of her father, and then the conclusion, "I think I have to go into [psycho] therapy, but I have mixed feelings about it. I'd like to find out how much of my trouble is physical." Her speech seems perfectly reasonable when put that way. The illogical, chaotic, "crazy" quality leaves it.

As I noted earlier, there were other facets of her speech (rate, pitch, and pausing) that made listeners think she was disturbed. When the speech rate was slowed, or the pitch decreased, she sounded normal again, despite the chaotic jumble of premises. Here I altered the logic to make her appear more clear-thinking, and again, she does not seem disturbed, despite the rapid-fire, high-pitched speech. Many factors in the spoken language play a part in our estimation of the speaker, but when one factor is changed or normalized, the effect of the others may be lessened. Here some features of her speech suggest to the listener that this patient is disturbed, but other features give the opposite impression, and the estimation of normality wins out. It is as though listeners try to give the speaker the benefit of the doubt.

In other settings, however, such as a psychiatric ward, the opposite might hold. The meaning of a speaker's utterances to the listener is influenced not only by what is said and how it is said but also by the context in which the utterance occurs. Sadly, even physically ill patients in emergency rooms are often presumed to be healthy when, if they presented their symptoms in the same manner, say in a private office, the fact that they are truly sick would be evident to the listener.

This patient demonstrates that a speaker gives the impression of being disturbed in many ways simultaneously: speech rate, pitch, pausing, word choice, and a chaotic presentation of premises. The impression of disturbance is also conveyed by a patient's manner of sitting, way of entering a room, choice of clothing, way of wearing it, and, in a hospital room, the appearance of the patient's bed and surrounding area, in other words, through the entire presentation of self. It is best to be aware of precisely why you perceive the patient to be disturbed, to make conscious note of all the verbal and non-verbal clues, so that your interpretation of "eccentric," "disturbed," "wacky," "nuts," "crazy," is made consciously, with your interpretation kept distinct from your observation of the data. (In time, as skill is gained, you may not be aware of what you saw and heard in coming to a conclusion, but, on reflection, the information can be returned to consciousness.) Note the informal language that I used to describe the conclusions. "Wacky," "nuts," and "crazy" are not very precise words, and to many they have a pejorative connotation. But our task is to figure out what to do for someone, and in the beginning of that task, a rough description points the way to action. For this purpose loose adjectives are much more useful than "paranoid schizophrenic," which is a diagnostic label requiring much, much more information about the patient than is available at this time. Using "eccentric," "disturbed," "wacky," "nuts," or "crazy" in thinking about a patient is much like thinking, in another context, that perhaps the duration and quality of the cough seems more lower than upper respiratory; this thought is not a diagnostic label but a guide for action, telling you to get a chest X ray. Unfortunately it is still difficult to use words like this in describing a patient to another physician, nurse, social worker, or other caregiver, who does not know you (or the patient) very well. They will usually think you are saying something bad about the patient instead of realizing they are hearing rough descriptive terms. If they paid attention to what you actually said, rather than making a value judgment about your attitude toward a patient, they would give more responsive care and learn earlier to dismiss, as irrelevant, categories such as "like" or "dislike" in referring to patients.

Hearing this patient's mixed-premise salad should alert you to search actively for the conclusion in her utterance. In addition it will warn you that the conclusion and the supporting premises may be difficult to sort out. Her opening monologue (in response to the question, "What can I do for you") lasted one minute and twenty-two seconds. This is a long time to keep in mind everything someone says. But the conclusion "I want to sort out what is physical" is quite reasonable. You are trying to find an entry into the problem, a handle that will allow you to begin. She has in fact given few symptom clues—unfortunately no symptoms were stated—that will allow opening questions. But suppose you were so overwhelmed by the presentation that nothing stuck? Knowing that there is always a logic, something that ties it all together, would prompt the question, "Tell me again, please, what is the problem you would like me to work on?" The patient will usually repeat her agenda: she wants you to tell her it is all the menopause (physical), so that she does not have to address her emotional problems. This gives the physician the opportunity to explore both sides of the equation and make appropriate recommendations or create the opportunity for further discussion. This procedure will help avoid those situation where, for example, estrogens are prescribed to solve what is essentially a drinking problem or severe emotional disability. It may equally avoid the prescription of psychotherapy when back exercises would do the job.

Let us return to the second example, provided in support of the everyday belief that speech is usually illogical or that patients are not logical. You may wish to go back to look at the entire transcript. The pertinent part is reproduced here.

Well, that pill wasn't for your boiler factory, that pill was for your blood pressure.

Well, I don't know what it— but this the— the fa—

You mean, the pill had that effect on you?

Yes, I wake up in a sweat. I didn't drop them altogether, but I took one like every other day, and I finished the prescription, and then I—

Now, when you took it every other day, did it give you that trouble at night?

It still, uh...Well, I felt I should take something to control my pressure, so once in a while I'll have a guilt feeling and take a pill. And then I took a couple from my husband's bottle, you know, he had the same. So, he was taking the medicine, I was taking the medicine, my son was taking the same medicine—I've had—

What's he taking the same medicine for?

For pressure— and I figured, well, one of us, we're gonna start looking for, uh, weapons— uh, who's gonna take the gun, who's gonna take the knife—

Well, you're all having the . . . reaction to it?

We're all upset—

What can that mean? Let us put aside the phrases that report her side effects. Then, after telling us that she takes an occasional pill, because she feels guilty at avoiding her medication, we learn that both her husband and her son are taking the same drug. For what? "For pressure." What does the word "pressure" mean? Physicians assume that "pressure" and hypertension are the same thing, that both words refer to the hydrodynamic pressure within the vascular system usually measured by a sphygmomanometer. But many patients equate the word "pressure," implying emotional tension, with the pressure measured on a blood pressure machine. The doctor asks, "Well, you're all having the..." but before he can finish his sentence, which refers to drug reaction, she answers, as though he were asking a different question, by responding, "We're all upset...." In other words, she is saying, "We are all taking the same medication for pressure. We are all upset." Now the reference to "whose gonna take the gun, whose gonna take the knife" begins to make sense. The next segment of that conversation was taped in the consulting room after the doctor and patient left the examining room.

Don't ask me why, doctor. (Crying) If you talk to my husband sometime, if you could indirectly ask him why he hates his son so much.

Oh ... That's what makes the unhappiness?

Very. He's killing me with it. I tell him it and he—I don't know, he just doesn't mean it I guess. He just does it. Just the way he acts, the way ... (sigh) It's just words, that's all, just words that are said, that make, that— the— they bother me, you know? ... My son isn't a child, he's forty-two years old, but, I mean, he's not perfect. No one's perfect. But he rides him all the time; every chance he gets he rides him.... That's just a little thing. There's no togetherness. See, now you got me all upset and get myself all teared up—not that it does any good. (Laugh) My problem is I cry too easy.

This is Aldomet, Helen.

Mm-hm.

One, twice a day.

Mm-hm.

If you have a problem with it, will you call me, please. I mean, all you do is delay getting your blood pressure under control, right?

Nothing— How could a blood pressure get under control when you always have aggravation?

The fact of dispute in the family has become clear. The premise, that the conflict between her husband and son is a source of emotional tension for this woman, is reasonable. Later she states the belief that it is impossible to control hypertension while emotional distress continues. What seemed at first to be a totally illogical outburst has become clear and reasonable. There are two reasons why the doctor failed to understand her; these are two reasons why the logic of a conversation may be obscured.

The first reason why the logic of a conversation may be obscured occurs frequently and was discussed in chapter 2. The listener hears the premise but attaches a different significance than the speaker to the words. With the *speaker's* meaning, the phrase makes sense; with the meanings attached by the hearer, the utterance sounds like nonsense. The listener, guided by the knowledge that normal utterances are always logical, must try to discover what has gone wrong. The most obvious method is to say, "I don't follow you, Helen, what are you talking about?" or "Please explain that to me." In this instance, since compliance with a regimen for hypertension is involved, clarifying the patient's misunderstanding is very important if her hypertension is to be controlled.

The further reason for failure to follow the patient's logical thread, in this example, is that the doctor was so involved in his own utterances that he seemed not to hear what the patient was actually saying, except for the fact that she did not answer his questions. Logic is to be sought not only in an individual statement but, more important, in the dialogue between speakers. When the patient's or doctor's utterances do not follow from what has gone before, then something has gone wrong. Failure to make sense of a patient's reply is a signal to restate the question or use some other device to clarify meaning. At the very least a loss of logical coherence in the whole conversation is a signal of misunderstanding.

Internal Contradiction: Being of "Two Minds"

Occasionally, when listening to a speaker, one hears every word, rearranges the premises, looks for the missing premise, checks for the possibility of misunderstanding or differences in meaning, and after doing all of these things, the conversation still does not make sense. This occurs because in some utterances there may be more than one logic going on concurrently. Consider the next example:

So, I-I really can't—

Otherwise you're well?

No. Otherwise I'm well. I have a wheezy chest that isn't the greatest chest in the worl-l-l-ld.

I've been hearing that. Now, while you're telling me you're well, you're wheezing.

Oh, wha— I am wheezing now?

Yeah, I can . . . . hear it.

I may be . . . . a little nervous now 'cause I'm talking to you and I'm—

Do you smoke?

No, I stopped.

And when does your chest get wheezy?

I can get wheezy on tension . . . I'll be perfectly honest, I can—Much of the time it is.

Do you get wheezy if you have a cold, too?

O— occasionally, occasionally.

If you have to rush along the street—

If— if I have a cold, and I get, you know, all the, you know, ickeyness with it, then I—

How many years have you gotten wheezy under tension?

Oh, years. I'll tell you what I do. It's a very funny thing. Under tension, I've reacted so queerly over the years. Years ago I used to get migraines.

Mm-hm.

But real stinkers.

Mm-hm.

For many years. You know?

Mm-hm. Now, ... when you walk along

But really—

the street, do you get short of breath from the wheezing.

I can—not from wheezing, but I'll tell you what I have done. I do get it if I'm going up—an incline.

—Up st . . . . . Mm-hm.

Otherwise, no.

So you get it if you goin'— You don't get it when you're washing or dressing though.

No, no, no. No.

Mm-hm.

If I'm in a hurry, or if I'm tense or I'm upset, I can— I can get a wheezing.

—hm.

I can get a shortness of breath.

Mm-hm.

Every—

And has that also been true for a long, long time—shortness of breath going up an incline?

Eh, no. I'd say that it's been true the past five or six years. But not for—

How many pillows do you sleep on?
One.
And you always slept on one pillow?
Mm-hm.
Do you ever wake up at night 'cause you're wheezy?
(Clears throat) . . . No, not really. No.
Do you ever get good, full-blown asthmatic attacks?
Uhhh, once or twice. Well—
What do you do for your—
—I had a little Tedral, and . . . I was fine.
How often do you take Tedral or anything for your chest?
Nothing—never do. I never take anything. Never find a need for it. I don't have anything, you know, in that sense that's bad enough—
Hm-hm. But, if you and I were going to race to the corner—
I might do very well! Now, I'm going to tell you something. I do better on r-running!
Mm-hm.
I can run and make a bus.
Mm-hm. Without getting wheezy or short winded?
Yes! Yes.
Does the weather seem to—affect your chest?
The wheeziness doesn't bother me nearly as much as getting out of breath. That— bothers me more.
Mm-hm.
When I do.
Does the weather seem to affect your chest?
(Sneezes) Uh, I haven't noticed it, no. I-I— my— weather affects my breathing, yes. That I do know. I can get clogged and blocked in very humid weather.
How about your breathing in here?
Well, if I get clogged and blocked, then I do get it, yeah.
Now, tell me about your colitis. 'Cause, you see, you're a lady without health problems, except you wheeze and you get short of breath . . . . . . when you walk up an incline.
I have a . . . yeah, I know . . . . Yeah, but I don't call those health problems. I consider myself very fortunate, but go ahead.

Is she well, or is she not? She is well. But she also has wheezing and exertional dyspnea. She has, by her own statement, a wheezy chest that is not the best chest in the world. She wheezes when she is tense and, occasionally, when she has a cold. She becomes short of breath walking up an incline. She has Tedral, which helps her chest, but she "never takes anything, never has a need for it." Even the weather, humidity, causes her to be short of breath. And at the end, she does not call those things health problems. Remember, the patient was wheezing while the conversation was in progress! The conversation does not make sense, if only because most listeners would think that she were describing distinct health problems. The conversation would be quite reasonable, however, if there were two speakers within the same body, and one were healthy and the other had chest symptoms. The patient uses "I" in referring to her symptoms and also uses "I" in considering herself healthy. It sounds like denial; it is at least self-contradictory. "Now why are you telling me you're well? You're wheezing." "Oh, wha— I am wheezing now?" In chapter 2 I showed how depersonalizing or distancing language might be employed by a speaker to diminish the impact of illness or symptoms. This example demonstrates another linguistic method for accomplishing the same thing. Before further discussion, a second example, which contains an enormous internal contradiction, will be helpful.

How much do you drink, alcohol?
Almost not at all. No big reason except I overreact to all drugs. All— everything. So I get drunk on one drink. That's why I drink very little.
Do you take any medication regularly?
Oh, boy, do you want a list?
Yup.
Okay. By regularly you mean on a daily basis?
Mm-hm.
Um, I haven't taken the Sansert in a long time, and I'm trying to go without it. And so far, I haven't had a recurrence of what...was diagnosed as "migraine equivalent."
Mm-hm.
Un, I take a grain of thyroid everyday—there's nothing wrong with my thyroid—
As thyroid?
Yuh.
Mm-hm.
There's nothing wrong with my thyroid according to all the tests. Metabolism was peachy.
Mm-hm.
Um, I take, ah, Actifed almost daily.

Mm-hm.

In the summer, more.

All right.

Um, sometimes vitamins. —I want to ask you about that later, whether you—

Mm-hm.

—believe in all that. And I take at night, once in a while I'll take a Valium in the daytime, if I'm having a very—pressured day. Um, the yellow.

What strength? Mm-hm. Five milligrams.

Yeah. Oh, ten, I go right to sleep!

Mm-hm.

And to sleep, I take, uh, five milligram Valium and a two hundred Noludar. And it works—a recipe of somebody's.

Together.

What? Together. They're low doses, and I've never had to increase them, luckily. Um, on a regular basis . . . Oh, I take Premarin now.

Mm-hm. What strength?

Uh, the ye— the yellow—greeny ones?

Mm-hm. One point two five.

Um, I think that's it. Oh, Probanthine, sometimes. That's my weak area. My—

Your stomach?

—stomach. Yeah, that's the place that gets upset the easiest and . . . reacts—

What kind of Probanthine?

—it's spastic, it's, uh, you know, all those things. What?

Is it the little shiny one or the long—

It's, um, the little pink round ones.

Mm-hm.

I think that's the list.

This patient overreacts to all drugs, "all—everything." The usual conclusion drawn from the premise "I overreact to all drugs," is "therefore, I take no (or few) drugs." Not only does this woman take several medications, but the doses (when we hear them) are not small. Thus listeners might conclude that the patient is contradicting herself.

In a dialogue we speak of there being a listener and a speaker, but in fact each pair represents two listeners and two speakers. When someone speaks, they may not always be pleased with what they hear, because the full, unpleasant meaning of their symptoms may only begin to dawn on them as they hear themselves answer the doctor's questions. It should not be a surprise when the part of them that has been avoiding the knowledge of the illness in the first place tries to mitigate the answers, to avoid the painful truth. But, to the listening doctor, it can sound like an annoying set of contradictions, an attempt to withhold information, to confuse, lie, or waste time. The patient in the next segment provides a prime example of this phenomenon.

I cough.
You cough.
Yuh.
Do you raise phlegm with this cough?
No. R-recently I have begun to raise a little phlegm, occasion— in the morning, occasionally.
And that's something new for you?
It's pro-gres-sive-ly more so. It isn't really, uh, . . . yuh, I don't do it all the time.
Mm-hm.
And it isn't a large amount of—
When you, uh— does your wheezing get in the way of your activity, your exercise, or— walking
No.
—up stairs, or walking— along the street.
No. No. No. No.
Mm-hm.
No.
And in this questionnaire, there are questions about getting shortness of breath when you walk—
Yuh, I— I ah, right.
Mm-hm. And did you—
It doesn't, really. I mean I— at the— at the time that I feel . . . that I—
Would you run up the subway steps?
I never— no.
Could you?
Yeah! Sure I could.
Would it stop you, your wheezing?
No, I don't— Look, I wheeze only from time to time.
Yes, but it's— Since you came back from September and certainly in the last week or so, you've wheezed enough so that your wife is gettin' up at night or— and—

She's got up from the coughing, not wheezing.
All right. Now, have you also wheezed during this period?
What period.
This period of the last week-and-a-half or two weeks.
Yes!
Right—And do you wheeze during the day?
Yes! (sigh) . . . I wheeze maybe . . . I— for a period.
Minutes period, hours period?
A period—I, oh, yuh. When I— when I— when I start wheezing
when I, you know, when I— (coughs) when I have—because then I
have a little trouble, you know, with my— with my breathing.
Mm-hm.
It's a good thing I'm not, you know, trying to sing at the moment.
Right. Mm-hm.
Uh, when I do, I— I take what I have been taking for—to control
hay fever, which is Chlortri— uh, uh, no, Pyribenzamine.
And does that help your wheezing?
It see— I think it does, yes.
*Right. Now, when—for how long, I'm now talking days—For how many days
has it been a good thing you're—*
Yes.
—not singing?
. . . . Oh, I would say . . . . a month!
Mm-hm. Now, when you were in South America,—did—
No.
you have—any wheezing—at all? Can you remember?
No. No. No! We were up at 12,000 feet.

"Do you raise phlegm with this cough?" "No," then "a little," then
"progressively more so," then "it isn't really," and so on, through the
interview. Another thing that happens here is that the patient does
not always answer the question. The answer does not logically follow
from the question. This is a rather common occurrence. "Did you
have pain again last week, Sam?" "Well, I'm eating much better."
But I did not ask about appetite, I asked about pain. A change in
subject is an attempt to avoid the question. Sometimes the subject
change is so subtle that it may go unnoticed. Other times the answer
seems to be to the same question, but a shift in wording changes the
meaning. "Are you taking your medication regularly?" "I try to take
it three times a day." To try to do something is not the same as doing
it.

It is difficult to discuss this phenomenon without becoming involved in attempts to explain it. Often the patient is accused of not telling the truth or actively trying to confuse the physician. I believe that, in giving a history, conscious intent to mislead or lie is not very common, although obviously it does occur; on the other hand, the phenomenon shown by these examples occurs frequently.

Perhaps the simplest explanation is that people can be of two minds about something: they can hold two conflicting points of view simultaneously. Even a very sick person might be of two minds about going to the doctor. Some do not like physicians, others are afraid of illness, still others do not like tests or needles, many have severe demands on their times; perhaps a hundred additional good reasons could be found for not wanting to be sick. Unfortunately, however, the patient's body is not well and demands attention, so the person reluctantly takes his or her body off to the doctor. Since the body does not have its own voice, the person is forced to report the symptoms and answer questions. It is little wonder that the part of the patient that did not want to come occasionally says things to counter the impression of illness—ergo contradictions that sound like deliberate evasions.

Doctors can only do their work by starting from the presumption that the vast majority of patients come to them in order to get better. I am well aware of the emotional, social, and legal "benefits" that illness can provide, but just as a cough is more often a symptom of a cold than of coccidiodomycosis, so the sick person more often wants to be better than not. Simply accepting that fact and leaving aside details of psychodynamics or moral behavior (that patient lied to me!), the physician can turn the occurrence of internal contradictions and inconsistencies to good use. The first step is to acknowledge that the two points of view represented by the conflicting statements are both legitimate. Or, put another way, the part of the patient that wants to deny the illness—not come to the doctor, not answer questions—or resist in numerous other possible ways must have a very good reason for being present in the patient, or it would not exist! The least useful course is to accuse the patient of lying, misleading, denying, or holding out. Getting angry at the patient is also (usually) counterproductive, since it further stiffens resistance and only provides further evidence to the resisting part of the patient that he or she should never have come. Thus the best response is to acknowledge the resistance as a legitimate part of the patient's behavior. "I know that the last thing you want to do is be sick or cough or wheeze, but . . ." or "I'm sure you have very good reasons for not wanting to be here, but

..." and so on. The "but" might be followed by "the quicker I can find out what makes you wheeze, the sooner you'll be well again," or "we just have to get through these questions. I may sound like the district attorney, but at least I'm on the side of the part of you that wants treatment." Another way of acknowledging the resisting part of the person is to use that part's own language in formulating questions. Note that the question that finally makes the wheezing man give some information borrows his own words to inquire, "For how many days has it been a good thing you're not singing?"

Accepting the concept that a patient may be of two minds can serve another function: this obstructing, denying, misleading "other" mind is nonetheless telling you about views held by the patient. The woman who overreacts to drugs can be expected to have a drug reaction unless she is convinced (both minds, that is) that she ought to be taking the medication you prescribe. This is, after all, what she told you. She may not have had a drug reaction, but you have been alerted to the possibility. The woman who is calling herself well at the very time she is wheezing is perfectly capable of doing the same thing over the telephone, thus concealing dire symptoms. Every patient in this group is capable of such behavior.

In summary, internal contradictions within an utterance may mean that the speaker is of two minds about something. Each of these minds can be quite logical and consistent, but when the two minds speak concurrently with one voice, what comes out may not sound logical. Both of these minds, or "selves," deserve consideration and careful listening. They are both legitimate aspects of that person, and they both have something to say that may be worth hearing. The doctor is sometimes the ally of one of the selves and sometimes of the other.

The Logic of Diagnosis

Another kind of logic to be considered is the diagnostic logic of the doctor. It is received wisdom that the history of an illness, in the patient's own words, is the most important source of diagnostic information. However, this underemphasizes the role of the doctor in the patient's storytelling. The process of taking the patient's history, even when you are listening attentively, is an interactive process: both doctor and patient participate. The value of the sick person's story develops not only through the narrative but also through the questions and answers that bring out the essential details. Although these details may be known only to the patient, the patient may not have been aware, prior to the questioning, of their existence and importance. Hence it is the doctor's trained inquiry that brings out the history of the illness. In the second volume of this book the process of taking a history will be examined in detail, but a few comments may be useful now. The doctor, in asking questions, has a hypothesis (the most likely diagnosis) or a number of hypotheses, which he or she is trying to test. The skilled interviewer is working just as hard to prove a given hypothesis wrong as to support it (in clinical medicine, as in the research laboratory, the null hypothesis is more easily provable). Each question aims to elicit, flesh out, or eliminate the premises necessary to conclude that some disease is or is not present, or that some action must be taken.

Here is a simple example. This patient came to the neurologist because of a persistent feeling of pressure in the head.

Have there been days during the winter when there was no pressure?
In the winter I have been going crazy with the pressure.
Have you been wakened at night by this pressure?
Yes. The pressure is very strong.
Do you have any nausea? Do you throw up?
Lately.
Lately you're . . nauseated?
Lately.
Since when? . . Since when?
I feel nauseous . . . . . This last two weeks.
Just the last two weeks?
Yeah, the last week, especially, this last week has been very bad.
. . . . . *Are you pregnant by any chance?*
No.
Is any of this pressure a throbbing pain, —like a pulse in your head?
It feel like if something pumping, do you mean?
Pounding.
Right. Right. In this side. In the left side. Always is the left.
Now, did you ever have any of this before, just once in a while, like migraine?
. . . . N-n-n-o, no before the year. Do you mean the pressure?
In the past?
No, never before. Yes, it just-a started a year ago, and since then I've been having this pressure and been going to all kinds of doctor for— for treatment to see if it's really physically, blood test, everything. They have done everything and didn't find anything.

The physician is accumulating evidence. His hypothesis is that the discomfort is due to increased intracranial pressure. Although he does not necessarily believe this to be true, this diagnosis is so threatening to the patient, it must be considered (the first hypothesis to be entertained should be the diagnosis that represents the most dangerous disease). If the symptom is due to increased intracranial pressure, then X, Y, and Z should also be true. Nausea, for example. Is she nauseated? Yes. If she is nauseated, does the nausea have another source? "Are you pregnant by any chance?" and so on. In the same manner the doctor goes after the throbbing sensation sometimes found in space-occupying lesions of the brain. He is orderly as he proceeds to flesh out each premise. I personally find this diagnostic process very enjoyable. When the problem is complicated and obscure and sickness threatens the patient, there are few tasks more challenging in all of medicine.

In this instance the patient's paralanguage strongly suggests that she is depressed. The sound of her voice is flat, with little tonal variation; her utterances are short, her pauses, very long. Of course she may also have a space-occupying lesion of the brain. The neurologist probably suspects her depression but continues working carefully to exclude a neurologic source.

Here is another example. This concerns one of the more elementary diagnoses but the process is the same.

Your last period was when? You —you had two or three normal ones, didn't you?

Right.

—Spontaneously.

Yes.

And when was the last normal one?

Approximately thirty-six days ago.

Was thirty-six days ago.

In other words, I think I'm about a week late.

Now, have you had any other signs or symptoms of pregnancy. For example, are your breasts tender? Do they bother you at all?

I don't—I wouldn't relate it—to that.

No. Any nausea or vomiting?

No.

Have you ever had urinary frequency? Have you noticed that you have to go to the bathroom more frequently, to urinate?

I do, but I don't that that it's—
So, as far as you know, you— you've really had no sp— no special signs of anything going on.
No, the only thing—
Okay.
—that we have not been doing is practicing active birth control—
Okay.
—other than withdrawal.
So, you've had unprotected intercourse since your last period.
Except for withdrawal and—
Okay. Let's take a look.

It is not a difficult diagnosis, but the questions must be asked and arranged in a logical pattern. Others, besides physicians pursue a logic of diagnosis; it is a characteristic way of making sense of the unknown. Listen to this woman:

Actually, for myself, I— at first I thought it was a pulled muscle, but then when it took so long to go away—
Mm-hm.
—then I was beginning to watch for like, a shingles kind of thing, you know—
Mm-hm.
And I thought, it just seemed to grow li— because it was spreading and—
Right.
—going across my back, and I thought, well, maybe it's, like, following a nerve trunk, you know?
Mm-hm.
I never saw any rash or anything, and—
When you get this pain, does it really grab you?
Well, well, no—
I mean, if you lie down in the wrong position, does it really get you like that, or— does it
No—
ache—or what does it feel like?
No, no . . . . no, when I will lay on my side after about three— I even timed it, you know, I found, like, five minutes was the longest that I could stay—I could stay longer, but that I was uncomfortable after five minutes.
Well, does the discomfort start the moment you lie on your side or does it begin—

Just a few moments after—
—and then it begins to build.
Shortly after. Yeah. And then it just—
And when it builds, does it build in intensity, in its extent, is it more and more part of you?
Yes, it seems to spread and it would seem— you know, get stronger. And . . . you know, I mean, it— it's nothing that was serious. I just felt like you just shouldn't have a pain in your si— You should be able to lay on your ni— on your left side without—
Mm.
—it being— having to move. And, uh, I—then I thought of neuralgia, and so on. I kept ruling out all these things, and then I began to think, well, what if it's something really serious and I—
Mm-hm.
—began to try to remember how you could diagnose Hodgkin's and all these—
Mm.
—various malignancies and . . . thought, "Is there something in my ribs or bones," and so on and so forth.

All of us have gone through a similar logical operation and come up with a malignancy, just as she did. She is a nurse, so her medical information is more sophisticated than the average layperson, but the process is similar.

This example raises an interesting issue that is intrusive in patient care. There is a premise hidden in this patient's conversation that seems to be universal, as true for physicians, when they are ill, as for everyone else. The premise is, "If I have a disease, it is fatal (or worse than fatal)." Cancer, brain tumor, multiple sclerosis, schizophrenia, or whatever dread disease is currently in the news, are the diagnoses that patients tend to apply to their symptoms. As we shall see, extracting symptoms from the maze of implications the patient has constructed is both necessary and (sometimes) difficult. I do not know why all people with sufficient symptoms foresee dire consequences, but they do. From the point of view of logic, there is no reason to assume the worst; quite the contrary. Since the "fatal premise" appears to be universal, the doctor must assume, until convinced otherwise, that the patient is either operating on it or defending against it (possibly through denial). Patients are often unaware that the "fatal premise" underlies their response to their symptoms. Surprisingly, telling them usually does not help matters.

Unconscious Beliefs

Unconscious beliefs, ideas, premises ("fatal" or otherwise), among other determinants of behavior, are unarguably present in everyone. They are called "unconscious" because they cannot be brought to awareness by simple recall. These unconscious premises are always operating to a greater or lesser degree. As a result we have to take for granted that part of the determinants of the patient's behavior and speech (and of our own also) that is inaccessible to our certain knowledge; it is open only to speculation, which may be more or less accurate, depending on our experience, intuition, or insight. Having said this, I feel justified in making my final point and asking listeners to hear what is stated out loud and then to act on that. A premise may mean what it says and twelve other things as well, but we can only *know* what is actually said. In fact one reason why it is so important to understand that all normal conversation is logical is that logic often suggests—given stated premises *A*, *B*, and *C*—that something as yet unstated must be the case. Knowing what someone has said then is an excellent starting place for discovering what they leave unsaid. Or, to put it another way, if you want to learn to listen with the third ear, the best way to start is to learn to listen with the other two. Indeed, sometimes a single word opens up the case.

The Pursuit of Clues

The next example shows the pursuit of a clue. It also shows how our understanding of a patient's speech is based on our knowledge of the world. This man, in his late twenties, came to the doctor complaining of an odd symptom—extraordinary sensitivity in his fingertips. Indeed, he could almost feel the energy of his plants growing. He had to stop working, because his fingertips were so sensitive he could hardly bear to write. It takes no acumen to realize that the symptom is, with high probability, psychiatric and perhaps even stems from an ongoing psychosis. The patient must be helped, however, and for this he too must recognize the psychiatric nature of his symptom. In the first part of the history no such recognition is present. On the contrary, the patient had fled a dermatology clinic when they advised him to see a psychiatrist. The sequence opens as the patient is being asked a standard question to elicit drug or other allergy.

Are there any foods or drugs that upset your stomach, make you break out, give you pain in your abdomen, or which you avoid for any reason?

Yeah, I don't like, uh, —I think it's Thorazine.

Why?

Tranquilizers. Because, uh, my skin gets very sensitive.

And when did you take Thorazine?

Uh, maybe two years ago.

Mm-hm. What was that for?

Uh, for some—uh—tranquilizers.

Th— thorazine isn't just like—

It's a tranquilizer.

—Miltown. I know what Thorazine is. What were you given the—

M-maybe it's not. . . . Maybe it's—

—Thorazine—

—not Thorazine. It's— it's a—

What did it look like?

They were very strong tablets . . . that, uh, that just made my skin very sensitive. I couldn't . . . go outside.

What do they look like—

They were little, round, sweet on the outside—

Orange?

Uh, th— that depends on the dose.

Mm-hm.

There were six hundred milligrams and three hundred and one hundred, I think, that I had.

Later, when asked about previous hospitalizations, the patient told about a psychiatric hospitalization. He virtually had no choice: the patient was aware that in discussing Thorazine in so much detail, he had revealed what was almost certainly a previous hospital admission for psychiatric illness. Thorazine, in the doses he mentioned, is most often an in-patient drug. With the previous psychiatric illness now a part of his known past, it became easier for the doctor to discuss the present symptoms in psychiatric terms. Let us examine the interaction piece by piece:

Are there any foods or drugs that upset your stomach, make you break out, give you pain in your abdomen, or which you avoid for any reason?

Yeah, I don't like, uh, —I think it's Thorazine.

The key word is "Thorazine." While Thorazine is an immensely useful drug in many nonpsychiatric situations, suppose this patient received it for a previous psychotic episode. How can the physician find out? If a direct question is asked, and the patient evades, by lie or other means (remember, he has already avoided the issue earlier in the history), the opportunity so essential to his present care is lost:

Yeah, I don't like, uh, —I think it's Thorazine.
Why?
Tranquilizers. Because, uh, my skin gets very sensitive.
And when did you take Thorazine?
Uh, maybe two years ago.
Mm-hm. What was that for?
Uh, for some—uh—tranquilizers.

It was taken, perhaps, two years earlier as a tranquilizer. But the patient has now heard himself, and his paralanguage attempts to minimize the word.

Th— Thorazine isn't just like—
It's a tranquilizer.
—Miltown. I know what Thorazine is.

The physician will not cooperate. Now, what was the Thorazine for? The patient establishes that he does not want to answer the question and attempts to backtrack. But the one almost certain premise is that it *was* Thorazine. Otherwise, how would the name have gotten into his utterance and then been identified as a tranquilizer? Now, the doctor, not only knows that the patient took it for emotional symptoms but also that the problem was, at least in the patient's eyes, major, not minor. How does he know? Because the patient attempted to conceal it. People rarely conceal unimportant things. If patients do conceal something that seems unimportant to the physician, it is not unimportant to the patient.

What were you given the—Thorazine . . . What did it look like?
M-maybe it's not— Maybe it's not Thorazine. It's— it's a—
What did it look like?
They were very strong tablets that—that, uh, that just made my skin very sensitive. I couldn't . . . go outside.
What do they look like—

Huh?
What do they look like?
They were little, round, sweet on the outside—
Orange?
Uh, th— that depends on the dose.
Mm-hm.
There were six hundred milligrams and three hundred and one hundred, I think, that I had.

It is unlikely that someone would casually know that much about Thorazine. The doctor then waited for the history of previous hospitalizations to emerge, to allow the patient to tell instead of appearing to force the information from him.

This next patient, who ostensibly came in for a routine physical examination, will reveal a serious symptom. You will see that his language telegraphs that he will reveal something. This is important, because when the symptom does arrive—angina pectoris—it is partly concealed. Once again, we are reminded that people can be of two minds about things. This man did not come to the doctor in order to hide this symptom that so concerned him. But, on the other hand (or, in the other mind), he would very much like not to be ill. In the odd mental calculus common to all of us, if he tells the doctor, and the doctor dismisses the symptom (easily accomplished if the doctor is not alert); then he is not sick! If you think this is childish, be more humble, because sooner or later in one area or another you will probably do the same thing.

I have really no complaints but I'm at an age where you need, once in a while, a checkup.
How old are you?
I will be sixty-eight in May. I have—I was thirty-two years in my job at C—— Records with—I never took time off for sickness except for an hern—hernia operation. And . . . I feel pretty good, but sometimes I'm a little bit . . . tired but I'm pretty busy, you know. Maybe this has something to do with it. I— I'm retired since two years, and I try to be as active as possible.
What do you do?
I'm on the staff of the Y—— University for recording operations—we built up some facilities. Then I did some teaching at the Y—— School of Music and now I do it at C——.
Mm-hm.
And the rest of my time is spent in a darkroom because I was very— much involved with photography.

Mm-hm.

And the only complaints I have, my—I filled everything out. I don't have any really—

Mm-hm.

I don't have any really— except if it's very cold, and I don't have a muffler on then I feel uncomfortable around the chest. Not that I have to stop, but it's just not—comfortable.

You mean when you walk along the street you feel this?

Yes.

If the wind is blowing on you?

Which—if it's very cold, and I am not warm enough.

How long had that been?

A year, two years, or so.

Mm-hm. Is it worse this winter than it was last winter?

No, much less.

Mm-hm. Does it happen any other time?

No—Maybe because I walked too fast uphill which I— I have no reason to do, really.

About how long you've had it—the walkin' up—uh—

Only I've had, really— really only if it's very cold.

Mm-hm.

—And then I have nothing. No more.

If you go up a flight of subway stairs—

It doesn't bother me at all.

Mm-hm.

Steps have never bothered me. I am European and am not scared of steps.

Mm-hm.

So, otherwise, I really have very little complaint. Once in a while— might be a little fast heartbeat which goes away. I take a deep breath, and then it disappears, and sometimes, uh, it may skip a beat once in a while.

When you say you have a fast heart beat, how fast?

. . . Not more than . . . maybe 110 or so.

Mm-hm. When will that happen?

Now that's a good question. . . . No—particular— When I get excited about something, I guess.

Mm-hm.

And very irritable, that's all.

Mm-hm. See, I ask like this because when you slip angina—by me like

Yah.

that, see, as though we're talking' about, you know, ingrown toenails or some-
thin', whe we really both know that although it— we— it's an important
symptom—uh—
Of course . . . . . Sure! Sure! That's why I mentioned all of these things.

The easiest way to clarify this example is to take it apart, step by
step. Before doing this, let me answer those who may think that in
analyzing the patient's logic in this manner we are making a mountain out of nothing. Remember, that this patient could have come in
and said as his opening line: "I've just come in for a checkup. I'm 67
years old, and I think I'm healthy, but it seems like a wise thing to
do." Remember, in each of these examples, there were alternative
ways of saying every phrase. It seems best to assume (again) that
people say what they mean.

Assertion 1   I have really no complaints
                 (*Premise: He is not sick.*)
                 Qualifier: but
                 I'm at an age when you need once in a while a
                 checkup
                 (*Premise: Just checking.*)
Question: How old are you?
Answer: I will be sixty-eight in May.

Assertion 2   I have I was thirty-two years in my job at C——
                 Records with I never took time off for sickness except
                 one hernia operation
                 (*Premise: History of health.*)
                 Qualifier: and
                 I feel pretty good
                 (*Premise: Not as good as possible.*)
                 Qualifier: but
                 Sometimes I'm a little bit tired
                 (*Premise: Not as good as possible.*)
                 Qualifier: but
                 I'm pretty busy you know
                 (*Premise: Actually he is fine.*)
                 Qualifier: I mean
                 (*Premise: He is unclear and unconvincing.*)
                 Maybe this has something to do with *it*
                 (*Premise: Something is wrong.*)

Qualifier: but
I'm retired since two years
(*Premise: He is okay.*)
Qualifier: and
I try to be as active as possible

Question: What do you do?

Answer: I'm on the staff at the Y—— University for recording operations... I'm very much involved in photography
(*Premise: He is active.*)

Assertion 3 And the only complaints I have ...
(*Premise: Something is wrong.*)

Assertion 4 I don't have any really
(*Premise: Nothing is wrong.*)
Qualifier: except
If its very cold and I have no muffler on, then I feel uncomfortable on the chest
(*Premise: Angina pectoris.*)

Angina pectoris. That is the way in which this diagnosis is made. By the time the symptom arrives, you, the listener, know it is coming.

This example makes another point. In the countless ways the meaning of words have been explained by linguists of different schools, the words that give the most difficulty are "but," "if," "maybe," "and," "or." They do not have referential meaning, like the word "typewriter," which refers to an object in the real world. They do not correspond to feeling states within the mind, like the word "worry," or abstract concepts held within a speaker, like the word "justice." We can see from the foregoing, however, that these words are logical operators, just as a "+" sign or "−" sign are arithmetical operators. They allow a speaker to stack premises together with "and," as though they were being added. One can qualify one premise by another by inserting the word "but," or give the premise an added meaning, using the word "or." Additional varieties and nuances of meaning can be imparted to the logical style of a speaker by other words such as "perhaps," "also," "necessarily." In the use of logic, as in every other aspect of communication, speakers can express themselves with ever finer shades of meaning.

The psychologist Edwin S. Shneidman has written on the logic of conversation in a most interesting manner. He has applied a sophisticated use of philosophical logic to examine the different styles of thinking displayed by speakers: what kind of premises they use, what errors in reasoning are consistently found in some and not others, and what means they use to turn facts one way or another. Using this as a base, he has attempted to define what psychological traits of the speaker are displayed in his or her use of logic. His work makes clear how much of value is to be found by a closer and more systematic study of the logic of conversation.

Putting the Logic of Language to Work

In these last two examples, particularly in the conversation with the patient who took Thorazine, we might picture the doctor saying, "I gottcha!, I caught you out, you sneaky devil," as though he were a detective who had just nabbed the bad guy. That is not the point: the point is not to see how smart you are. The point is to find out what is the matter with the patient and help him or her return to health. Helping patients achieve the maximum function of which they are capable, within the constraints of fate, is what doctors should be doing. This is why we listen to hearts and to chests and why we should listen to patients.

In this chapter, however, the curious phenomenon of people being of two (or more) minds about their symptoms, their health, doctors, medical care (and virtually everything else), has surfaced. The physician may be working for (and with) one part of a person—one "self"—seemingly in opposition to another. The fundamental assumption of medicine is that the mutual relationship between doctor and patient is inherently benevolent. They are not adversaries. The examination of the logic of conversation, with all that it can reveal of the symptoms, beliefs, assumptions, and premises of patients, is a tool that helps serve this relationship.

References

Schneidman, Edwin. The Logic of Politics. In *Television and Human Behavior*. Ed. by Leon Arons and Mark A. May. New York: Appleton-Century Crofts, 1963.

4

What Do People Mean When They Say What They Say?

This chapter is about two separate but related subjects. What is the intent of the speaker, and how credible is what has been said?

These are crucial issues. I have stressed the importance of hearing every premise, every paralinguistic feature, every word, as the basis for understanding the speaker. But suppose the speaker's intentions are not honorable? Suppose the patient is lying to you, or cheating, or trying to wangle a prescription for narcotics? In such instances the patient's words would have little diagnostic value. Suppose, on the other hand, that all physicians were engaged in trying to extort money from patients. If this were the case, then patients would be unable to interpret the physician's intentions, and his or her speech could not be used as a reliable guide to action. Indeed, if such base intentions were the rule, then the techniques I have been expounding would have no value.

Some physicians do in fact perceive patients as deceivers. They take an adversarial view of the doctor-patient relationship, as though patients were out to withhold the truth from them or otherwise do them damage. Unfortunately the enormous number of malpractice claims in the present era has reinforced this view. In addition all physicians in training have had the experience of spending hours trying to obtain an adequate history, and then having someone else obtain the crucial fact from the patient. They are sure the patient withheld that information from them on purpose (when in fact it was due to their own inexperience). A few moments' reflection will show how difficult it would be for a physician to care for the sick if they were all viewed as adversaries, as enemies trying to get something they do not deserve. But whatever your view of the relationship between doctor and patient, that viewpoint will be crucial to your assessment of a speaker's intent and credibility, and your knowledge of intention and credibility are basic to your understanding of that speaker.

Therefore, as part of examining the problems of intent and credibility, this chapter will, of necessity, deal with some aspects of the doctor-patient relationship.

Credibility

Some definitions are necessary. *Credibility* is defined here as the reliability of a speaker's words. What is the truth value of a statement made by that speaker? If the patient says the pain started the day before yesterday, is that when it started? "I used to weigh one hundred and twenty pounds, and I lost ten pounds." Does the utterance compare well to objective reality? Did the patient lose ten pounds or eight or twelve pounds? The problem presented by spoken information is more serious in medical practice than in ordinary conversation. Because error can be dangerous, when we ask when the pain started or how much weight was lost, we need to know the degree to which we can trust the information given.

Ordering a laboratory test poses the same requirement for accurate information. When the serum T-4 comes back 5.3 (normal is 5.0 to 8.4), does that mean it is normal? In fact the T-4 assays done by the laboratory that I use have an accuracy of plus or minus 14 percent. This means that a T-4 of 5.3 may represent normality or hypothyroidism. Some laboratory tests are much more precise than others. For example, no laboratory would report a white blood count as 14,350.6. The method is not that precise. However, the number after the decimal point, in a weight of 76.5 kilo obtained by a hospital scale, is perfectly reasonable. In addition to the concepts of accuracy (how well the measurement corresponds to the thing measured) and precision (the degree to which successive measurements differ from each other), much has been written lately about specificity (the number of false positives) and sensitivity (the number of false negatives) in tests and measurements. These concepts have helped to make physicians aware of the fact that a test or measurement (everything from oral temperatures through blood glucose levels to coronary angiography) is "true" only within certain limits of confidence. All reports from the laboratory, the X-ray department, indeed from all sources of medical information, are probabilistic. They have a certain probability (sometimes known, as in the T-4 that is "correct plus or minus 14 percent," but more often not known) of being correct; virtually nothing is the "absolute truth." Nothing is certain.

In the same way information acquired by listening to what patients say or by questioning them is "true" only within certain confidence limits. It has a certain probability of being correct. The concepts of accuracy, precision, sensitivity, and specificity apply not only to tests and measurements but also to what patients tell doctors about their bodies, their symptoms, themselves, others, events, and relationships. The reliability of measurements is affected by the methods of investigation. A better method produces information that is more accurate, more precise, and a better predictor of whether or not a disease or other state is actually present. A better method narrows the confidence limits and increases the value of information in probability terms. This is equally true of information obtained by listening to patients. This book teaches better methods for obtaining reliable diagnostic information from patients by speaking with them.

Intent

Knowing the intention of a speaker presents greater problems than determining credibility. *Intention* is defined here as a person's reason or purpose with respect to speech, what the person means by a statement. It is the split that occurs in the "meaning" that creates the problem of intent. The split is between what *the person* meant by what was said and what *the words* themselves meant. For example, if I say, "It is raining outside," the words mean if you look out of the window, you will see that it is raining. But what I meant when I said this was that you should put your rubbers on. Here the literal meaning of the words "It's raining outside" is different from the intention of the speaker, which is to get the listener to behave in a certain manner. Thus one of the obvious reasons that a listener cannot know the intentions of a speaker for certain is that words and sentences do not have intentions, only persons can have intentions. Words are used, however, to convey intentions. Words can be perceived; they are "things"; and one can prove they existed. Not so for intentions; they can never be known, measured, or their existence proved, in any objective fashion. Intentions are irreducibly subjective—they totally and completely depend on their possessor.

The Linguistic and Philosophical Problem

The problem of the intent of a speaker has driven linguists and philosophers of language to distraction; they cannot answer the "simple" question of how one knows the intent of a speaker. The reason is as simple as the question. No one, not even a speaker, can be certain of the speaker's intent. Behavioral psychologists sidestepped the issue by avoiding reference to the inner states of persons—desires, purposes, as well as intentions. Instead, only observable events were considered relevant to psychological description. But the problem of intent cannot be made to disappear by wishing it away. Philosophers of language tried seeking intention in the actions represented by the words. For example, the phrase "I promise to come to dinner" contains its intent in the verb "promise." Similarly "I pronounced the patient dead" contains its intent in the verb "pronounce." This system works fairly well as long as one stays with relatively simple utterances. It breaks down with the more complex language that characterizes natural conversation. Classical linguists sought intention within the structure of language, but this also failed. While I have oversimplified the positions taken in these approaches to the problem of intent, it is not an oversimplification to state they are attempts to avoid dealing with the mind, inner state—call it what you will—of the speaker. But as the psycholinguists have made clear, to find the intent of an utterance, you must go beyond the words. Words do not have intentions, speakers do.

The Medical Problem

Let us then go beyond the words and find an approach to the problem of knowing a speaker's intention that will work in the arena of medicine.

Our perspective on the problem of intent is special because of the unique relationship between doctor and patient. This is, in many ways, a very odd kind of relation between people. For example, in New York City there are people who consider me their doctor, although we have never met. In the address book by their telephone, entered under the word "doctor" is my name. They have been given my name by friends and consequently know something about me. They do not go to physicians often, and so years may go by with me as their family doctor despite the fact that they have never seen me. Then one August day they need a doctor in a hurry, and I am away on vacation. I have failed them. I have never met or spoken with them, but I have failed them. And they become annoyed at me. On the other hand, I may have cared for someone during an illness in 1967 and then not seen him again until 1977. During all those years the relationship between us continues. When the patient visits my office in 1977, we start up a conversation as though we had seen each other regularly all those years. There are friendships like that—

people one seldom sees with whom friendship requires no renewal—but such relationships are uncommon.

I remember a patient, lying undressed on the examining table, who said quizzically, "Why am I letting you touch me?" It is a very reasonable question. She was a patient new to me, a stranger, and fifteen minutes after our meeting, I was poking at her breasts! Similarly I have access to the homes and darkest secrets of people who are virtual strangers. In other words, the usual boundaries of a person, both physical and emotional, are crossed with impunity by physicians.

These unusual features of the relation between doctor and patient lead us to two additional characteristics which are crucial to understanding the intent of a speaker in a medical setting. First, it is inherently a benevolent relationship, and second, an intent is itself a fundamental part of the relationship. The sick patient comes to the doctor to get better. This is what the relationship is all about. (I am aware that patient and doctor may have vastly different ideas of what constitutes "better" and that considerable negotiating may be necessary before they can agree—if they ever do—on a common goal; this, however, does not change the basic intent of the relationship.) Doctors are with patients not to sell them stocks or talk about automobiles or argue politics but to make them better! I cannot think of another conversational setting where the underlying intent is so solidly preestablished. In street conversations, cocktail parties, or most settings where people talk to each other no consistent preestablished underlying intent is present, except for the basic rule of conversation that one intends people to understand one's words. This particularity of medical communication makes it easier to examine the problem of intent.

There is another aspect of the doctor-patient relationship that must be discussed, when examining intent: the expectations contained in the role of "physician" and that of "patient." Patients have the right to expect me to be warm, dignified, kind, open, trustworthy, giving (and forgiving), gentle, and perhaps to embody other characteristics usually associated with someone whom we love, or who is a parent, but not usually associated with strangers. The role of physician involves an obligation to behave in this fashion, even when my stomach is upset or I am angry at my spouse. Moreover I am obliged to extend myself in all these ways to many different people day in and day out. Clearly it would be impossible to give of oneself constantly in this very personal fashion without being pulled to pieces. Rather, doctors express kindness, empathy, warmth, trust, and all the other important characteristics, but it is not themselves they are giving. It takes quite a while in the course of training to learn (and some learn better than others), but we physicians do not lose a piece of ourselves when a patient dies or gain when one is born. This is a way of saying that the role of physician has not only obligations but also limitations. There are things that patients are entitled to receive from a physician in addition to technical knowledge, but there are also things to which they are not entitled. The converse is also true. There are also things to which physicians are entitled because they are physicians, but there are limits here also. Obligations and limits are a part of all rule-governed human interactions, from marriage to the law courts. Our concern is how this aspect of the role of physician and that of patient affects the problem of knowing the intent of the speaker. The effect is great. If a patient lies to me when I am taking a history, the patient has not lied to *me*, Eric Cassell. People are not supposed to lie to one another. A lie is like cheating, it is a moral offense. The medical setting changes this. The patient has lied to *the doctor*, and in that context the lie has a different meaning. Instead of being something done to me, the lie, once discovered, is a piece of information that can be used to help care for that patient.

The same thing applies to seductive behavior. When the patient behaves seductively, it is not *me* that is the object of seduction, it is *the doctor*. And so it is with anger and fear and a whole host of human attitudes and behaviors. Often the word "transference" is applied to the behavior of patients with physicians, but the term has acquired so much ideological baggage that I prefer to avoid it. My central point is that the way a patient behaves toward physicians is a part of that patient's relationship to illness and medical care. Fear of physicians may express fear of the body, of disease, or of painful treatments. All this is important to know when you take care of a sick patient. Illnesses are individual because persons are individual. This individuality is expressed in relation to the physician. And this relationship can be read, in part, through the intent of the speaker's word.

You may think that all I have said is that doctors should not make value judgments about their patients, no matter how the patients behave. I mean more than that. Whether the patient intends to (say) deceive, seduce, intimidate, or conceal, this behavior should not be taken personally or judged in moral terms; instead, the behavior should be considered medical information. These are facts about the person, as the heart murmur is a fact about the heart. Liars are different kinds of persons from nonliars, and extremely honorable people are different kinds of persons from less honorable people. In addition a patient who lies or deceives once may well do it again, and this is necessary information for good medical care.

Thus, when the doctor listens to someone talking and asks inwardly, "Why is this person telling me this?" "What does it mean?" the doctor is looking for medical information. The particulars of language by means of which such assessments are based—how people talk, their word usage, their logic, their presumed intent—are particulars in diagnosis and treatment. They resemble white blood counts, electrocardiograms, urine sediment, T-4s, heart murmurs, or palpated abdominal masses, with the problem of reliability being the same for all of them. "True" information is obtained only within certain probabilities.

This next example will bring us full circle:

Are you taking all of those pills?
I certainly do, yeah.
Two and one every day and one every day and one when—
One— one at the end of every other day—
—you have to.
—and one every day.
Yeah . . . Are you taking the heart pill?
Yeah!
Big one.
Every day.
Uh-huh. Why—
And the other one I take every other day.
Uh-huh.
Yeah
And the other one twice a week.
Yeah, the— the fluid pills—
The water pill.
Yeah, yeah. That's the one.
Take two.
Two what?
The one you take one every morning.
The big ones?
Yeah. The big ones. Take one in the morning and one at night.
One in the morning and one at night.
Yeah.
Oh.

Not the one you take one every other day, it's—
No, no, no, I'm not.
—the other one.

The interchange is a model of obscurity. And yet the importance of knowing what patients mean when they tell about their medication is undeniable. The importance of clearly telling them what to take, and how to do it, is equally undeniable. This little dialogue might be more than amusing; it might be fatal. In this example, however, the central problem is not the intent of either speaker, but what was meant. The intent of the physician seems clear enough: he wants the patient to take "all of those pills." If this is his purpose, however, then we realize that an intention is not clear unless the meaning of the language conveying the intention is clear. Or, put another way, if I intend something, if I mean something to happen, then one measure of clarity is whether or not you understood my intention. Intentions may be more than generalizations, such as "I want you to take medication." They may be as specific as, "I want you to take .25 mg of digoxin every morning before breakfast, and I also want you to take 40 mg of furosemide on alternate days in the morning, at the same time as the digoxin, and with one tablespoon of potassium supplement." If there is uncertainty about the directions, then the intention was uncertain. There are of course limits. The point here is that the intention includes the speaker's purpose, not just the meaning of the words. Intentions can be general or extremely specific. The same utterance can convey one or several of the speaker's intentions ("Take this medication," as well as "See how much I care," as well as "See what a smart doctor I am").

These complexities of the issue of intention are what have so challenged (paralyzed might be a better word) students of language. Knowing the intention of the speaker, however, is so vital to attentive listening in medicine that we must find a way around the problem. Moreover, despite the fact scholars have been confounded by the problem of knowing the intentions of a speaker, five-year-old children seem to have little difficulty with it. We can be sure little children have solved the problem, because they usually know what you mean when you speak to them. If it is so impossible, how do kids do it? I think that children know what you mean because, in common with all other (nonscholarly) speakers and hearers, they "know" (although they may be unaware of the knowledge) that one cannot know the intent, or meaning, of another with certainty. If we begin by accepting that fact, then the problem of intent is transformed into the problem of uncertainty.

How do speakers and hearers deal with the problem of uncertainty? For us physicians this problem should be of particular interest, since uncertainty is our constant companion.

Figuring Out a Speaker's Meaning

What the Speaker Says
Let us start with the kind of evidence listeners use to help them figure out what a speaker means. The first kind of data are what the speaker says. It is obvious, as I pointed out earlier, that the words and phrases may convey meanings that differ from their literal meanings. "Yes" is not the answer to the questions "Do you have the time?" or "Can you pass the salt?" You can think of many phrases that have acquired meanings that differ from the actual words. If you respond to their literal meanings, you may drive others wild and be thought a bit odd. Thus, whatever words mean in terms of intention, they do not always mean what they say. There is a contrary fact about them: words mean precisely what they mean. They may be used to convey numerous intentions, but the words mean what they mean. Because of this, words, which seem to be "just words in a meaningless phrase," sometimes send a message of which you are not aware. For example:

Um, let me introduce you to the first-year class, Mrs. Grace, and as I mentioned to you, I'm just going to sit and chat with you a little bit about, uh, about some of the, uh, the problems. Would you tell us about, uh, the troubles that you've had and that brought you to the hospital?

When the physician says, "Can you tell us about the troubles that brought you to the hospital," what is he saying? Generations of medical students have been taught to say "What brought you to the hospital?" as the opening in taking the history of a hospitalized patient. And in every group to whom it has been taught, some wit has said, "The taxi," because the literal meaning of the phrase requests the conveyance. But what we mean is, "Tell me about your sickness." The patient generally gets the idea, but patients also hear what the doctor actually said: tell about the "what," it interests me more than the "you"; you did not come to the hospital, you were brought by the "what" (the illness); you are passive to the illness ("what"); since I am interested in the illness, you are passive to my interest. These are the sets of meanings suggested by the phrase. Most physicians, certainly most teachers of medicine, would object to these meanings. The whole trend of modern medicine is away from such a harsh interpretation of the relative position of patient, illness, and physician. If they do not mean this, why do these physicians use these particular words? I take it for granted that people say what they mean. Even if the usage is initially only careless, the doctor who is saying these words also hears them, and after he or she has said them often enough, then that *is* what is meant. Here is another example.

What has been the problem that's brought you to a neurologist?

A problem did not bring her, she brought the problem. There are, after all, other ways of saying the same thing. "Why did you come to see me?" which is rather simple and direct. In my office I use "How can I help you?" with its several meanings, all intended. Here is an opening for a hospitalized patient with a long and complicated illness.

When— when were you last entirely well?

The words "what brought ..." and "chief complaint" (what the "what brought ..." is suppose to elicit) all come from medicine's musty past. We would do well to let all those tired phrases rest in the past. They have served us well, however, if they illustrate that words can carry nuances independent of, and even contrary to, the speaker's intentions. The meaning of words cannot be only idiosyncratic, known in the special way that you use them only to you, or they will have lost their utility to convey meanings to others. This next example comes from my office.

You know, each of the examples that you gave— They're all frustration examples.
Yeah.
You have no frustration tolerance.

Virtually every person who has heard this example believes I was criticizing the patient because she has no tolerance for frustration. I was not. Rather, I was trying to underline what seemed to be the essence of her symptom, as she had explained it to me. It was an aspect of her fatiguability (secondary to hypothyroidism). From my point of view it was a clarifying statement, but she also took it as though I intended criticism. The meaning of words is not only what you intend, it is also what has been heard as their meanings. We all have had reason to object, "But that isn't what I meant." One of the features of the spoken language is that the generally accepted meaning of utterances is their meaning, and a speaker cannot arbitrarily decide to use the same words to serve another purpose and expect to be understood.

The Social Rules of Conversation
The meanings of some phrases are established not only by linguistic conventions but also by social rules of conversation. If I ask "How are you?" as the opening statement of a conversation, it would break a social rule for you really to tell me. We all recognize that this is not a genuine request for information. The next patient, who was literally dying (and looked that way), describes what happened in her back yard:

I'm not much for talkin' though.
What are you going to talk about?
No, I mean with the neighbors.
Uh-huh. Well . . .
The neighbors talk to me, wave to me, and so on.
Are you comfortable . . . . most of the time?
You see, my houses . . . . are connected.
Mm-hm.
And if I go out in the yard to do the least thing, there's people out there—
Mm-hm.
—you know, and you have to talk to them. You have to say, "Hi." They say, "How are ya?" And, you know, you'd say, "Fine," or, you know, "Doing good," or "Going slowly," or "Doin' nicely", . . .

No matter how sick she appeared or felt, she was required to answer in this way. Now that all patients have telephones by their bedside and can be dialed directly, they respond with "Fine thanks," even if they will be dead within the hour. These patients never say "Dying," or "In agony," in response to the salutation "How are you," that would be a breach of rules whose force is enormous.

Sociolinguists studying the first few minutes of conversation have demonstrated that the order of speaking and turn taking in conversation are also governed by strict social rules. It has been stated that the relative social status of speakers determines who speaks first, so that the physician, who has high status, usually says the first words.

This does seem to occur in a doctor's office. The patient enters, and the doctor starts the conversation with "Hi, how are you?" and then the patient answers. In a hospital room, however, the patient usually says the first words when the doctor comes in. This would suggest that relative social status is not the only determinant of the order of speaking. Perhaps it is a territorial matter. It is the doctor's territory in the office and the patient's, in the hospital room. Whatever the reason, the rules are strong and are not easily breached. When the rules are broken, this lends a special meaning to the conversation. In this next example I break every social rule about speaking to another adult, while talking to a man who is ten or fifteen years older than I.

...goin'. Now, come on—

Mm, mm, mm, mm.

—I'll tell you. This—

Mm, mm.

—is what this all comes about and listen carefully to me. All day long people have been trying to get you to cough—

Hm, mm.

We're not ju— playing this whole game, going to lose it because you won't cough, I'll tell you that.

Oh— (mumbling)

And I really mean it. Too much work and too much worry. Now start coughing.

...Oh...

We'll produce—I'll tell what I'll do. I'll trade you a bowel movement for some real coughing.

mm...

And I will, I promise you that bowel movement.

Naaa—

I mean it. I promise you the bowel movement—

I—,

—but I want coughing.

Uhn—

Come on.

Uhn-huh, uhn-huh...Unh, uh, uhn...

Come on, cough—

Uhn, uhn, uh-uhn-uh—

—breathe

Uh-uhn-uh-uhn—

Blow, Nat.

—uh-uhn.

Blow on my hand.
(Sound)
That's not blowing. BLOW.
(Sound of blowing)
Harder.
(sound of blowing)
Now breathe in . . . Blow.
(Sound of blowing)
Breathe in.
(sound of inhalation)
Now blow out and breathe in again . . . Now . . . what do I see?
Okay.
Now, you're not moving your chest when you breathe. You're trying to keep your chest—
Uh-huh.
—from hurting. And while that's very understandable, the problem is that it just fills up with all kinds of crud— and, if you can't cough it out yourself, then it's going to be suctioned out.
I've been coughing it out myself here during the day—
Never, you— I'm sorry— sir, you have not . . . You can't bargain with this—
Mm-hm. But you gotta take it easy.
No we don't have to take it easy.
No you're not going to suction me.
Oh, yes we are!
No you're not.
Oh-ho, surely we are.
O-kay. I been doin'—I tell you, I've been doing my level best—
Well, your best isn't good enough so we'll suction you. That'll do it. We'll just suction him.
No more—
No, no, no.
Give me a rest, gimme a—
No, there's not rest 'cause the thing is there. You want to rest? Rest now. Now you rest. Put your feet down—put your shoulders down, and let yourself back into that pillow. Come on, you can relax. This is like having that other tube in, Nat.
Well, count me out.
Count you out?! I don't think we will.
Uhnnnn.
Yes, it really is the case, Nat. Tomorrow is a much better day. This is just somethin' you have to get over with.
Let me explain— (cough)

Cough! . . . Cough!
(coughing) You don't understand. You guys won't let me talk
. . . You're really a bunch of bastards.
That is the truth. You got it. That is the absolute truth. We are bastards.

One is conventionally not allowed to speak to adults in this fashion. The conversation thus achieves much greater force precisely because of the shattered conversational conventions, and this force emphasizes the underlying intent. He (and everyone else at the bedside) knows that the yelling and swearing are because of the intensity of my commitment to get him better.

In the same manner, when the rules are broken by the patient, this tells the attentive physician that something is wrong, even when the content of the conversation is relatively routine. The most obvious example is the panicky patient on the telephone who does not say "Hello" or "How are you" but plunges right into a description of the symptoms. The urgency in that situation is expressed as much in the breach of rules as in the utterance. This next example, taken from Patrick Byrne and Barrie Long's study of doctor-patient communication in England makes the the same point in a most poignant manner.

Good morning. Come in, Mrs. . . . Lynch, isn't it?
. . . yes.
Now, then, you've moved to Rochdale, it says here.
Yes. I moved yesterday but . . . but I'm back.
Back?
Well, I don't like the house there.
Where, uh, where are you living now?
Where I was before.
Oh, I see. Wh— now, what can I do for you?
Well, that's why I'm here . . . 'cept I'm not a' tall where?
. . . *Yeah* . . .
Where, you know . . .
What?
Where . . . they said I-I should come and see you about the pill.
Oh, the pill. Is that what you want?
Wel— ca— can I have it?
Oh, sure, but, um—I mean, have you spoken about this before? Let me see . . . there's nothing here on your card. Let's see, you're, um, how old? You're

thirty-seven and you have . . . no children. Uh, why is it that you want the pill? What are you doing at the moment.

It— it's not for me, it's for her.

Who?

Mrs. Davis?

Mrs. Davis?

She-she lives next door.

But I don't think she's my patient.

Oh . . . Well, then, I-I'll have my tablets then.

Tablets?

Y-yes, you know, th-the yellow ones. Pills.

Ah-huh, Valium. Oh. You know, we can do that whole thing by phone. If you just came here for— for a prescription we ca— I can call y— you can call me, and I'll call th— the pharmacist. Uh, so, ne— here, you take this, and next time you can— we can do this over the phone.

Okay. 'Cept, can I show you this?

. . . Christ! Where did you get that?

Well, he had done it last nigh when I walked out.

How long has it been bleeding?

Since last night.

Sure, let's get that cleaned up, huh?

You'll not tell the cops, will you?

Tell the co-—Wh- why would I do that?

Well, I-I thought you had to i— every time you see something like this.

Not for something like this, no.

's good. He hit me with a sheet of glass.

A sheet of glass?

Mm. Threw it as I was leaving.

Well, we'll have to get you to the Emergency Room. I'll have my secretary make the arrangements and, uh, you'll be there in five minutes.

(Byrne and Long 1976)

In the early part of the interaction, the patient did not do what a speaker is supposed to do: state her business. Parsimony is one of the rules of all conversation, and especially so in a medical encounter. The woman did not, would not, tell the physician what her trouble was, and many doctors find such behavior very annoying. Every person who comes to a doctor has a reason, however, and if the reason is not obvious, the physician must discover it. This is especially true when the reason for coming has been obscured by the breaking of conversational rules. Fear, or more often embarrassment, make people evasive. A response that is more effective than a show of impatience or irritation is to say: "I'm sure something must really be bothering you or you would not have so much trouble telling me; I will do my best to help you." The speaker is not doing those things to *you*, he or she is acting this way in *the doctor's* office. The doctor just happens to be you.

Sometimes a listener can hear the words, not understand them, and yet can understand their intent.

Okay, Mrs. Bronsky. You're going to have to have an EKG.

A knee KG? My-my knees okay. When it rains they hurt but this is . . . no trouble, you understand?

Uh, uh it's— no, it's connected to your heart.

Huh?

You don't understand. An EKG is connected to your heart. THAT's why we do it.

'knee KG?

You got it, that's what I'm saying.

Knee in the heart? . . . Ah, it is news to me . . . You're the doctor!—

The patient did not know what an EKG was or why she required one, but she understood that their intent was in her service.

What the Listener Knows about the Speaker

Another way hearers understand the speaker's purpose is through their knowledge of the speaker. My wife, a student, a colleague, and a patient may all say the same thing, and I will attach different meanings to each utterance, depending on who said it. I remember reading that investigators had attempted to study natural conversation by recording the language of married couples. The researchers gave up in despair, because they could not understand what the subjects were saying; no one finished a sentence! My wife and I usually know what the other is going to say well before the sentence ends. We understand each other's meaning and intent, which is why the words can stop in midsentence.

Many of the examples used in this book are from interactions where both participants had previous knowledge of each other, sometimes for years. This next example could only come from two people who know each other.

Marvin

Yes, sir.

Now listen to me. Let me tell you something . . . Your problem isn't your diseases— Your problem is not your diseases. Your problem is you're driving yourself crazy . . . It I—I'm not asking you—I never tell you, an-and that you' never hear out of me: "Listen, what do you expect, you're so old," or anything like that. You'll never hear that from me. And you'll never hear me say, "Accept" anything. "You gotta learn to accept it." I'm not telling you that. But I will tell you this: that when somethin's better, you gotta put it down! Now, your head is so much better, and yet you don't let go of it. Your gout is much better, but you've got another thing. —Marvin, you're dying from dying! You're not dying from diseases. . . .

He has told me about his diseases, but I am responding from what I know of him. Similarly what he understands me to mean comes from his knowledge of me as well as the words. It is our knowledge of the individual person that allows us to say: "Oh, Joyce didn't really mean that." "What do you mean, she didn't?" "Oh, I know her, and that's her idea of a joke." "Some joke!" Someone says something, and they think it's the funniest thing they ever said. But you sit silently, crushed, wounded, as the speaker touches the one sore spot that people who know you never talk about. The next example was the beginning of a discussion about sex that was, ultimately, very important to this patient.

I have some dumb questions to ask you, too, so—
Ask dumb questions . . . That's what I'm for.
Yeah?— Oh, oh. Okay. (Laughing) I'd like to ask you a dumb question like, is there a primer book on, on the physiogomy or whatever you call it, of the human body?
Yes. About . . . . what part of the body?
There is? Like the part that's engaged in intercourse.
Sure—D-d-t— tell me more what the que— what motivates the question.

Another patient might have said: "Do you know a book about sex?" and I would have produced a title. I knew this patient to be extremely shy, however, and the question, which I started to answer literally, was really intended to open quite a different conversation. The "real" question, the one intended, was "Will you talk with me about sex?" It is obvious that, in the same way the listener knows the speaker, so too, the speaker knows the listener and shapes the words to portray the intent to that specific listener. Feeling the same need, the patient might have posed the question differently to another physician.

What we know of a particular speaker is important in understanding his or her intent, but also important is what we know of the class of speakers. Physicians spend much of their lives being dealt with not as the person they are but as a member of the class called "doctors." In social groups they become accustomed to hearing everyone's "doctor story" when their profession becomes known. "We all know about doctors (lawyers, accountants, teachers, Indian chiefs); they always ..." This is stereotyping; it can apply to professions, social classes, racial or ethnic groups, or gender, but the effect is the same. The listener will hear the speaker and interpret the intent and meaning of the utterance more on the basis of the stereotype than on the actual words. While often such stereotypic interpretation closes the hearer's ears to the particular individual speaker, there are unquestionably racial, ethnic, class, and professional differences that influence the meanings of a speaker. It is not bigotry to recognize the effect of culture on individuals. It is foolish, however, to allow that knowledge to override what is actually said. Any effect on meaning that you believe comes from the "class" to which the speaker belongs can be confirmed by questions; it should no more be presumed to be true than presumed to be untrue.

This next example typifies reactions to physicians as a group.

You got an office someplace else? Someone told me. You got your own office?

Yeah.

You have? Where?

...Somewhere.

Oh, boy, that's a great answer. Y-y-yeah, oy, not supposed to tell, eh? 'Cause sometimes I say, "Ask my friend to come to the office."

...It has nothing to do with here. You can come.

Yeah. Well, if you say "somewhere," it can be on the moon. (Laughs)

(Laughs) But it has nothing to do with here.

No. You're at your PRIVATE office.

Yeah?

Yeah, good!

Tenth Avenue, Seventy-fourth Street.

Really. Well, it's nice—it's nice to know, if it should be closed or something here.

Tenth Avenue, Seventy-fourth Street.

Tenth Avenue and Seventy-fourth Street...But it's outside the Clinic, right? That's why—

It's nothing to do with this Clinic.

No. No.

Over there, I'm a different—

Yeah. Boy, you have some business then. Huh?

... What do you mean, "You have some business?"

You—well I mean, I-I, uh, maybe I shouldn't say it like that. I should, maybe, you are—you must be quite busy, you know, be—

Yeah.

—cause you work in here, work in— That's what I meant to say.

Yeah ... Okay.

Here is another example of a reaction to physicians.

The problem really is this: um, I've been to two different endocrinologists and, in both cases, nobody'll TELL me anything! And, um—

What do you mean they won't tell you anything.

They won't tell me anything. It's like—

They must tell you SOMEthing. They must—

—you, know, they go, "mmmmmm" or "Hmmmmm" ...

Do they—

I-it-it's like you always get the feeling that you're sort of getting the bum's rush out of the office and you never know the difference.

"Everybody knows about doctors ..." When the person opposite you has that running through his or her mind, you may believe it is not you, the individual, who is speaking and being heard. People do not usually speak as "the class of," they speak as themselves. But if you wish your words to have their intended effect, you must be aware that the listener may be so strongly influenced by the stereotype, that your words are ignored.

The Listener's Knowledge of the World

People's knowledge of the world at large is also used to help them understand what a speaker intends, and the plausibility of the story told.

I have a nice big sink, and I have beautiful drapes, and I haven't seen one roach.

Not a single roach, huh?

Not one. And remember how many there were in the hotel—

Mm-hm.

About a billion. .... Not one.

Were there any other animals?
Yes, and they do speak of a lion.
They speak of a lion?
And I had to pass it in order to avoid trouble and— Doctor, that wasn't funny (laughing).
Walking by that tail, you mean?
No, it wasn't— every time I went by, the tail went like this, you know— (laugh)
Was it in somebody's room?
Yes. With a girl—
Mm-hm.
—who lives, um, who went away on Friday, and she didn't come back 'til Monday, and she was there, and she went to sleep on the same pillow, and she developed a terrible disease. She had terrible lumps all over her face and her body and her legs.
Mm-hm.
And I told the hotel that she ought to be examined—
Mm-hm.
—and she did leave the next day.
Where do you think she got the disease from?
From the lion.

This patient is schizophrenic and actively hallucinates quite commonly. I do not believe there is a lion in that hotel. The knowledge of the world used to interpret a speaker's meaning grows with life experience. Physicians are fortunate that they are exposed to, and can learn from, the life experiences of so many people. I encourage patients to tell me about their work and their world because it gives me the opportunity to learn more about people and how they live. The more I know, the more I am able to understand of what they tell me. It can be said truly that everything a physician learns about virtually anything is part of his or her medical knowledge since, sooner or later, the information will play a part in the care of the sick.

In the next example we will first hear the wife talking and then, separately, the husband, followed by both together. Her reason for not wanting another anesthesia is that she developed an amniotic fluid embolism following the birth of her last child a year earlier and was mortally ill for quite a while.

What kind of birth control do you use?
Uh, what right now? Withdrawal...I don't want to get into my— my birth control. That's another whole story, but, uh—

Well, now—

So—

Can I—so you don't have any bir—

Well, I'd like my husband to have a vasectomy, and we've been discussing it now, and I know it's a—

But, what at the moment, is—you're gonna do until he has a vasectomy and maybe—

Well, this is—

—he doesn't want to have a vasectomy.

Well, this is the thing we're discussing.

Why don't you have your tubes tied?

Because I don't want to go in for another operation. I don't want to be put under any kind of anesthesia again.

Now it can be done without your—you know in— the point is that vasectomies and tubal ligations are very—are things that are not like cuttin' your fingernails.

Well, that's why we're—well, that's why we're not having it done.

You ever heard of a diaphragm?

Yeah. Well, this is—I was going to go and have it done, and this is what we're doing in the meantime—

Doesn't this sort of get—

I don't like t—

—in the way of your sex life, Kathy, if you don't mind my being nosy? And I'll tell you I am.

Yeah, I—it does. But, you know, sex is not a major part of our relationship, and right now, withdrawing is no major problem for him.

Okay.

———————————

Our knowledge of the world causes us to doubt the statement that "Sex is not a major part of our relationship." Further most of us would think that withdrawal is a poor contraceptive method for several reasons. We would suspect that sex and birth control have become a problem for this couple. Her husband had come with her to see me, and this next segment occurred while he and I were in the consulting room waiting for her to dress. (He was not wearing a microphone but was recorded through mine.)

———————————

Now, I wanted to talk to you about the subject of birth control . . . I think my wife mentioned it, and, uh . . .

Well, she mentioned it, and I discussed it quite a bit.

It's really a problem.

Contraception . . . You're not happy with the kind of contraception you're using now?

No. Not at all. It's a problem.

I'm gonna discuss it with her briefly again, 'cause it came up, and I took it up. That's—the kind of contraception you're using in your house right now is not considered the world's best of all the contracept— It makes for unhappy people.

Mm-hm.

Our suspicions are confirmed. In the next conversation we are all together in the consulting room.

I want to talk about one other thing which is not my area except your husband brought it up.

(Laughs) Birth control.

Yes. These are areas where people live. They're not necessarily areas that they talk about, every feeling they have about it, but it's where people live. Sex may not be a big thing in your house, lady—

(Laughs) Sorry I said that. (Laughs)

From her embarrassed laugh, we know that she too realizes a problem exists. In the previous chapter on logic we might have said that her explanation for why they use withdrawal for contraception does not make sense. Her premises are not credible; on the basis of what we know about men and women, sexuality, and young couples, we do not believe what she says. Further her intention in choice of contraceptive method may have to do with other issues, such as anger at her husband which may play a part in why she wants him to have a vasectomy. These are speculations; they can be confirmed in further discussion if this should be necessary and appropriate. Here we discovered the problem by interpreting her meaning through our knowledge of world. What we knew of the world suggested that what we were hearing was very odd.

Self-Knowledge

Part of the knowledge used by listeners in interpreting the intent of others is self-knowledge: what the listener would have meant if he or she had produced the utterance. What it feels like to be burned . . . what an anesthesia entails . . . how hot it is in New York City in August . . . how it feels to suffer from tourist diarrhea . . . how difficult it is to swallow large pills . . . , all of these and an infinite number of other facts and feelings are part of an individual's knowledge, not only from hearing or reading about them but through direct experience. The same kind of information shapes the meanings people assign to events, objects, or relationships. Such knowledge allows a listener to interpret what the speaker means. This type of interpretation generally occurs without the listener being aware of the source of the information, although it can usually be brought to consciousness. The errors in interpretation that arise from the listener's assumption that the speaker shares the same intent and meanings may not have serious consequences in ordinary conversation, but they can cause major problems in medical interactions. On the other hand, the benefits of such assumptions to the attentive listener may also be considerable. When I am in doubt about the meaning of a symptom report, I attempt to elicit the description of pain or other symptom to the point where I can *actually almost feel the physical distress*. I remember seeing a patient who had been told that the chest pains of which she complained were angina pectoris. The discomfort—low substernal, lumplike, and tight—did not sound as though it were cardiac in origin, but I did not know what it was. I asked her repeatedly to describe it. Then in the examining room, as I was about to examine her fundi with the lights out, I suddenly knew what it felt like. Grief or loss of a loved one produces that feeling: a sad heaviness in the chest. This allowed me to ask some more questions, which confirmed that she was losing a long-standing, beloved partner. But it was not until I could almost actually feel the discomfort that I discovered its source in her, and I could not "feel" it until she had described it over and over again.

Sometimes, having experienced the disease or distress yourself makes understanding easier, as the next example suggests.

But it left me with this noise in my ear.
What kind of?
A noise like a radiator is always "sssssssing", you know, like the radiator's steam comin' up. That's—
Yeah.
—always. It just sounds like steam coming out of your ear. You ever hear of steam comin' up out of a right ear? That's the way it sounds. And then, whenever it— but once— sometimes it's worse than other times. And if you run the water, it isn't too bad; you hear the water runnin'; it overcomes the noise.
Uh-huh.
When it gets real bad at night, I get up, and I take a Valium, and then I put on the water, and then I know that I'm all right, you know. I go back to sleep from the Valium, but not from—it doesn't to the— i-i-

it, that doesn't cure the ear. I often worry about having stroke from it, you know, I—

Well, I don't think, uh, it has any relationship to strokes.

No, that's— that's the best part of it. When you know that. Believe me, unless you have a, a good doctor that explains it to you, and if they just shake their head and say, "You have to learn to live with it," you feel like saying, "You don't know what I'm talking about."

Yeah.

There has to be somebody— I happen to have been very lucky. I had a man, a da— a doctor, who was, uh, robbed in the office. And, at the particular time I was having the trouble, and, uh, there was a shot fired in the office, i— in where the doctor was—not when I was there but before—and the doctor was left with tinnitus so he had a lot of sympathy for me.

Yes.

From the shot.

Yes.

So he knew what I was going through, you know. And, so, I had— then I had a lot of faith in that doctor 'cause he knew, (laughing) he knew what it was, you know?

It was not until I developed asthma that I realized that coughing may be the only symptom of bronchospasm at some periods of the illness. Repeatedly asking about wheezing will not only *not* reveal the diagnosis, it will also make the patient wonder whether you understand. The physician who, by continually asking questions, learns what things feel like to the patient will be be better equipped to find out what actually is the matter and will confirm that he or she understands the patient. This comprehension will be genuine. To know the intent of the speaker is, in the most simple terms, to understand. Understanding is a very complex and poorly delineated concept, but it is a vital component of an effective relation between doctor and patient. It is not necessary to acquire every disease that your patients may have (although it might be useful), but it is desperately necessary that you try to comprehend what they are trying to tell you. The patient who believes that you understand will more often do what is prescribed and probably get better faster. Part of the intent of an utterance is what it tells you about how important something is to the speaker. The woman telling the doctor about the ringing in her ears intends that the physician know, not only that she has tinnitus, but also, how important—how distressing—it is to her. To empathize with her is to understand not only the factual implications of her words, but also the importance to her of what she is describing. This is another situation where we must be very careful about what we say. In questioning and requestioning, the physician should communicate a desire to comprehend, rather than the possibility that the patient cannot be understood. As always, everything the physician says has special meaning to the patient, and a careless utterance is not permissable.

The Speaker's Presentation of Self
One intention of the spoken language, hidden or overt, is the presentation of the self. Almost every utterance contains something of the person of the speaker. In earlier chapters we saw how the person is present in word choice, paralanguage, and logical usage; here, these things come together. Listening to discover the purpose of the speaker's utterance is also listening to discover the speaker. Sometimes speakers present themselves in more than one way at the same time, as in this next example.

Have you ever had any operations?
....Oh! I had plastic surgery six months ago—
For what?
—my first operation. I had a little minilift.
And you're pleased with it?
Very pleased.
Okay.
It was my first operation. I'm pleased except for one thing which you'll see onto—it's the doctor's fault and he admits it. I got two giant hematomas, and he did beautiful surgery. I— went and had a— I had a revulsion against the whole idea. I mean, it's one thing to go to Konoffsky and, um, earn a slim body and good muscles; it's another thing, passively, to be cut and made prettier. You know, I really found it repugnant.
Mm-hm.
Then a girlfriend of mine did it and then she sort of paved the way for me. Um, and then I thought, 'Well, it's silly not to'...

This is the same patient as in chapter 3, on the logic of conversation. There, she implied that she could not take medications, because she was so sensitive to every drug. Then she rattled off a long list of medicines she took regularly. Here, she admires the idea of self-improvement while finding "repugnant" the idea of plastic surgery. But she had the plastic procedure, which she minimizes by calling it a "little minilift." She is pleased with the result, which was "beautiful surgery" . . . except for . . . And that is the surgeon's fault. One might, without fear of contradiction, say that she is of two minds about her surgery. Things are both beautiful and not quite right, best achieved both naturally and by means of medical techniques, done because she so chooses, and, at the same time, causing difficulties which are the fault of others. Has she not told the physician about herself? Or rather, about both "selves?" Which "self" will emerge, when she is ill and recovery is slow and painful? The overwhelming probability is that slowly resolving illness, or even an episode of low back pain, will bring out the impatient, negative, fault-finding woman.

On other occasions the speaker's presentation of self is direct, as in this next example, where the man speaks in the measured, cadenced tones befitting his statement of self.

. . . No, first of all, I— Look, I'm not the kind of a fellow that wants to hear you pat me on the back because, uh, while I'm an egotist and recognize a lot of things, I have a lot of faults because I'm an uneducated person. I use the word uneducated because, uh, maybe I— there are certain things that I lack. Uh, at best, I'm a high school graduate. That's all. I've gone very far in the field of finance and economics with men who hold high degrees; I sit around with men who count in this world and they recognize my little talent that I have, and when I say recognize, they count on me to go and do things. Unfortunately, I'm too devoted to my clients and to my business. I can't help myself. If you said to me, 'Irwin, I have this house on Se— Sixty-ninth Street . . .'

Seymour has presented himself. The knowledge contained in the utterance was ultimately crucial to his care, during a hospitalization in his final illness. Doctors often spend much of their energy helping sick people preserve themselves as the persons they are. Yet the skills necessary to help patients effectively maintain control over their own worlds, remaining as much as possible the persons others recognize as authentic and whom they, themselves, wish to be, are unfortunately not a part of the manifest training of physicians. As a result doctors have to acquire such knowledge experientially. This is a pity: some will never learn, others will do it poorly, and for the rest of us it is an inefficient and slow way to acquire these crucial skills.

Seymour was in the hospital with end-stage cirrhosis of the liver. Reducing the massive ascites and edema which necessitated the hospitalization was a slow process. One day he said he had to go home. It seemed inappropriately soon to me. He reeled off, as the reason for leaving, a litany of complaints about the hospital. After bargaining for a while, I said he could be discharged on Sunday. "I have to go home on Friday." Why? He needed more than one day to rest up. For what? He wanted to go to work on Monday! Sick unto death, he would go to work, where he would be with the important men, who recognized "his little talent" and counted on him; where he could be himself. We found a way for him to go to work. If I had not responded to that need in him, he would have signed out of the hospital, and compromised his treatment even more.

The point is that his "self," the person he felt himself to be, was crucial to his treatment. Recognizing that self required no magic, he described himself directly, in simple language. You will rarely have only one opportunity to hear who the person is, because the self is presented as part of utterance after utterance. Sadly, many medical listeners brush off the part of the utterance in which the self is found, in their eagerness to get at the "important" content, relevant to the disease. But it is the person *plus* the disease that makes the illness which the physician treats.

The Context of Conversation

Another kind of evidence that helps a listener figure out what a speaker means is the context in which the words occur. It is obvious that words have different meanings depending on the setting of the conversation. The word "setting" implies this, insofar as it recalls the theater. It is the scene that creates the mood, so that by the time the actors speak, the audience will hear the characters themselves rather than people acting parts. Imagine meeting somebody on the street who said, with a straight face, "What fools these mortals be." He or she would sound like a fool and a pretentious one, at that. Meanings and intentions have a quality of seriousness, or weightiness, as one of their dimensions. Clothing and general appearance can be considered as part of the context of a conversation. Certain dress is appropriate for one profession, or occasion, and not another. Thus bankers look like bankers; if people try to speak as bankers while lounging in pajamas, they test the credibility of their listeners. We can all think of more intimate situations where these rules apply. The rules apply as much in medicine as elsewhere. The emergency room, the operating room, the waiting rooms, all the settings of the hospital, add (or subtract) meaning and weight from the speech of everyone involved. Doctors wear white coats and may have stethoscopes in their pockets: all the world knows they are physicians and that their words carry messages of life and death. When I was a student, I wore my white coat with pride and hoped my stethoscope dangled with just the right nonchalance (I knew more about wearing it with style than hearing anything through it). All of these contextual features emphasize the meaning and importance of the doctor's words, helping the patient accept the otherwise unacceptable.

It is important to realize that context is as important to the listener as to the speaker. Thus, when physicians dress too informally or otherwise disregard conventions of personal appearance or speech, because they feel they should have complete freedom in such matters, it is not themselves alone that they influence. In matters such as their health and safety, patients require the additional assurance that context adds to the words of their physician. Television and movies employ appearances, dress codes, and settings to transmit intents and ideas to the viewer much faster than if each meaning had to be stated explicitly. Meaning and intention are transmitted with the same speed in our daily life, where context influences the way listeners and speakers respond to one another.

The History of an Utterance, an Interaction, a Relationship
Fragments of conversation, even whole conversations between others, are often difficult to understand because of the fact that every interaction and every phrase in an interaction has a history that contributes to understanding the moment. This history includes what the speaker has just said, the way the speaker uses the social rules of conversation, what the listener knows about the speaker and class of speakers, the listener's knowledge of the world and self-knowledge, the speaker's presentation of self, the context of conversation, and more. One reason natural conversation is difficult to study is that utterances and conversations do not float free; the history of the utterance and the relationship between the speakers enable the listener to figure out the speaker's meaning. Let us examine a brief utterance taken from a conversation between an oncologist and his patient, recorded in her hospital room.

"I'm ashamed of the people, already."

What does that mean? Literally, it means that she is ashamed by what the people did (or are, or seem). This is what she says. Here is her phrase and the doctor's rejoinder:

You stay here, okay . . .
Oh, I'm ashamed of the people, already, that I'm not home.
Why? Wh— ashamed for—

I don't know.
—*What reason? You're in a hospital, you're not—you're not goofin' off. That's ridiculous.*

She does not mean that she is ashamed of what the people did, she is ashamed of herself! Ashamed of what the people will think, because she is still in the hospital. This is not what her words said, but a listener processing her phrase in milliseconds—her doctor actually cut in before she had finished the phrase—knew what she meant and responded appropriately. This is the miracle of spoken language. I looked at her utterance, printed on a page on the wall of my laboratory, for months and months, trying to figure out how her doctor could possibly interpret her phrase correctly in that short time. The answer did not come until the entire conversation was heard. I am going to present it here with some interruptions for explanation. See how much redundancy there is; how each theme is played and replayed. You can think of the conversation as a sonata, in which a few major themes are brought up and then elaborated. As presented, it is six minutes long (nothing has been left out except for the few minutes while the doctor was examining the patient's chest and abdomen). The exchange could be condensed to a minute or two without the loss of any important content—but then, it would not be conversation.

Now, now I don't know whether you'll like this recorded. I suffered something terribly—
I heard—

He enters the room, and the conversation, with an expectation: the conversation has a history. Theme 1 is "I suffered terribly," and the staff has already told him that.

—today.
I heard.
I cannot—
Stomach?
—go on like this— stomach. And then it went to the back. I just couldn't move.
All right. They ta— I talked with them. I think this is probably the medicine. I'm not—
I know.

—going to let you go home on Saturday. I've already talked to the doctor that's here on the floor. I'm going to keep you through here, through next week.

Ohhhh, through another week?

Theme 2 is the possibility of reaction to medication, and theme 3 is about going home. All of the themes have been mentioned within the first moments of conversation.

Now, now I don't know whether you'll like this recorded. I suffered something terribly—

I heard—

today.

I Heard.

I cannot—

Stomach?

—go on like this— stomach. And then it went to the back. I just couldn't move.

All right. They ta— I talked with them. I think this is probably from the medicine. I'm not—

I know.

—going to let you go home Saturday. I've already talked with the doctor that's here on the floor. I'm going to keep you through here, through next week.

Ohhhh, through another week?

Well, I gonna keep you— Tuesday at least. —well, I— I'm going to be away Monday and Tuesday. Dr. P——r will be here, but I don't think we want—

Ohhh.

—to quite let you go home as long as your stomach is giving you all the . . . trouble that it's giving you.

(sighing) Ohhh.

Okay? So, it—

But I'm wond—

—It may be from the medicine. You've got to have the medicine, you understand.

I understand, but I must have a little relief in between.

I'm going to give you something to try to get you to— Did you move your bowels all right today?

Yes. I have no trouble moving them.

But you still have a lot of cramps and pain.

Yes, but mostly pain, pain and cra— It woke me up at four o'clock this morning. I sleep—very little.

With the cramps? —All right, let's take a—

—as it is.

—Let's take a look and see that we got here . . . Now show me where you— Put your legs up flat, sweetie . . . Now show me where most of your pain is.

This way.

Going up here?

Yeah— but on the side, this way. Both sides.

Does it come around the back this way here?

Yes, it comes around the back.

And it comes over this way, this—

Yeah.

like this. What about on this side, same—

This side—

thing?

—same thing.

Does it go down into your crotch, so to speak?

No.

All over this way?

Yeah.

And does it come up from the back around here?

Yes, it goes into the back.

On both sides?

Both sides.

Uh-huh. And you moved your bowels okay.

Fine.

All right.

They look at them every day.

Are you having the pain right now? No.

Mild.

Right down—

Right here.

—here. Yeah. This all looks like toxicity from the—

Yeah. Yeah.

—medicine. Any tingling in your fingers?

No,

Not a bit, huh?

No. A little numbness once in a while.

A little bit but not a whole lot.

No,

Okay. Take a deep breath . . . . again . . . . deep . . . And you never had a problem like this previously?

No,
Not until the medicine started.
I—No, I had—I used to have stomach cramps. The whole thing started with cramps.—
All right. Now—
—and then I had a barium enema taken—
And—
They found nothing.
Nothing.
I had—
When was the barium enema done?
In, uh, early September ... at Dr. Z——r's.
Of this year? Dr. Z——r.
Yeah.
And also, what about the upper GI?
Normal.
And when was that done?
Same time.
Uh-huh. And the gall bladder was done, too—
Same time.
And everything was negative?
Negative.
All in September.
Yeah, except the chest X ray which showed water in the lung.
You already had the water back in September as I recall, isn't that right?
Yes, I think that was the last X ray he took.
Uh-huh. Then they tried to get you in the hospital here, I guess—
Yeah, Dr. Mc——e got me in, yeah.
Okay. All right. So, um, did they x-ray your kidneys?
Uh—
What they call an IVP.
Yes! Here.
Mm-hm.
I had it.
Mm-hm.
Mm-hm.
But you're having this from both sides, not—
Yeah

—from just the one side.
No, both sides. That's not the kidney. It—
—I—
—feels like the muscle.
I— I think this is, uh— have you had pains like this before that responded to Donnatal?
Yes, it responded, uh— I had cramps that responded—
Is it— is it the same type of cramps that you're having right now?
No.
These are . . . different.
This is a———different type.
Different. How are they different?
Because I get it mostly on the sides here?
Uh-huh. Where was the cramps that you were having before? Up higher?
Yeah—yah. In the center.
Uh-huh. But the same—
Right.
—sort of discomfort?
Not as bad as now.
Not-as-bad-as-now.
No. No.
All right. Well, let's see. And you're moving your bowels okay.
Fine.
When did you have those other cramps that responded to Donnatal? Do you recall how long ago that was?
Yeah. That was in Aug— last August.
August a year ago.
The doctor gave me C-Cantil. You know what Cantil . . ?
Mm-hm.
Cantil. And Donnatal. And-d uh d-uh, I had bad cramps, and she told me to take, uh, Darvon—
Mm-hm.
—but she forgot to tell me to, uh, be x-rayed.
Mm-hm. But in— in any event, uh, that worked very well for you.
On and off. On—
Uh—
—and off.
But you said—
But the cramps disappeared.

Uh-huh. But now you got 'em back for—
Yeah.
—the first time.
Yeah.
I think this is mostly from the medicine we—gave you.
Oh, I'm—sure of it. I' sure of—
You didn't have these cramps 'til I started giving you the medicine—
That's right.
All right.
That's all right.
Well, let's hold off on— on the medicine. I'm going to start another medicine on you in the meanwhile, but I'm going to hold off on this one until—
What d'ya mean, you're going to hold off on the cortisone?
On the Vincristine. No, you're going to get the cortisone. I'm going to hold off on the Vincristine which I think is responsible for this. I'm going to start you on some medicine, uh, uh, this week. And in the meanwhile we'll wait and see what happens with your stomach. If your stomach gets better through Monday and Tuesday and Wednesday I may give you a much smaller dose of the medicine. See, it makes me very hesitant—
Yeah, but will I get in the meantime for relief?
I'll give you something. Does the Darvocet work very well for you? Darvon work for you?
No, not too good.
Well, I don't want to give you anything too strong 'cause it'll just constipate you, you know?
Well, Darvon is constipating.
Yeah. See, the thing is I don't want to give you a whole lot. I don't want to give you anything too strong. What about— we'll try—I'll give you those. Let me try—Have you ever had Talwin? Does that make you upset?
Uh-uh- I had Talwin when I had the tube inside of me.
Did that help you?
No, not with the tube in there. That was very painful.
No. But that— this isn't anything nearly as painful—
No.
—as that. This is just more rumbling in there.
No, it's more than rumbling, it's deep pain.
Mm-hm. I just don't see very much here right now.
No, I don't feel anything when you touch it.
See, when I push here, you don't have very much—
No, no.

This is mostly, I think, a little bit of ileus associated with the Vincristine. Maybe we'll just stop it, and I'll just start on something else and we'll start to reduce the cortisone on you.

And when— well, will that— will, will the fluid come back in my lung?

No, I'm going to start something a little bit different. I hope not. No, I'm— that's what I—that if we get some fluid back—

That's what I'm worried about.

No, no, no. Let us, let us do it our way. Okay? All right, now, hold on—

No, now another thing. The sleeping medicine that I take doesn't work very much any more.

All right.

I sleep only about two hours.

Well, I'll change that around. That's no problem. Okay?

I take the, uh, Darvon and the Nembutal . . .

All right.

It doesn't work very much on me. And this thing woke me up, I got crazy during the night.

Okay. Well, I'll see if we can give you something, uh, to make you feel better—

And—

—but stay here next week. There's no hurry. You stay here.

Oh, I'm ashamed of the people, already, that I'm not home.

Why? Wh— ashamed for—

I don't know.

—what reason? You're in a hospital, you're not—you're not goofin' off. That's ridiculous.

S—

So let's keep you here through maybe Wednesday or Thursday and then we'll let you go—

Oh, boy. Another week.

Well, I think it's better.

I think so, too.

All right.

Uh, Dr. Cohen, will you do me a favor?

Sure.

My daughter's very anxious to speak to you. You want her telephone number?

Yeah, sure.

She's there now, if you want to call.

All right, I'll be glad to give her a call.

See the amount of repetition about the nature of the abdominal pain and its relation to bowel movements. The issue is vital, and the doctor works to make sure the information is in fact what he thinks; she too works to make sure the doctor hears her viewpoint and symptoms. Notice how knowledgeable this woman is about her lymphoma, the medications, and diagnostic studies. She is representative of the modern patient. (The days have gone, I am glad to say, when the doctor can get away with simplistic, kindergarten explanations.) This woman has information and needs information.

By the time the phrase, "I'm ashamed of the people, already," enters the conversation, there has been so much conversation about going home that the doctor could hardly fail to interpret the utterance correctly. The miracle of almost instantaneous processing of meaning loses its miraculous quality within the context of the whole conversation.

Listeners understand the speaker's purpose by the meaning of the words (including paralanguage, syntax, and logic), the social rules of conversation, what the listener knows of the individual speaker and the group(s) to which the speaker belongs, the listener's knowledge of the world and of self, and by the context and history of the conversation.

Yet after all these sources of information are brought to bear, the listener still cannot be certain of the speaker's intent: The young man sat in the apartment of his beloved, and she said, "Darling, I love you more than anybody in the world. I adore you. But, I have some things to do, so please go home now, and I'll call you later. I love you." Overwhelmed because of her words, the young man left reluctantly. On his way out of the building, he saw another young man heading for her door, and suddenly the meaning of her words changed: she was trying to get rid of him! The point is, one can never know the intent of another with certainty. Everyone knows this; it is part of social life. Consequently everyone comes to accept an irreducible level of uncertainty. Speakers and hearers, however, have evolved methods to reduce uncertainty. Such methods may be one of the primary reasons for the marked difference between spoken and written language.

Conversational Mechanisms for Reducing Uncertainty

Substituting the Listener's Intent
The first method for reducing uncertainty is when listeners bring their own intent to the conversation: they hear the meaning and intent

they want to hear. Consequently the listener's needs and purposes are used by the listener to extract meanings pertinent to these needs from the speaker's utterance. The classic example is the "double take"— sudden recognition of the true meaning several moments after an utterance. The double-take illustrates that the listener did, initially, hear what he or she wanted to hear; later the words "percolate" through the set of expectations, and a second interpretation is made. The next example comes from the first office visit of a man who had an episode of neurological disease with aphasia that occurred while he was in college. It was initially thought to be psychiatric illness, and he was sent to a psychiatric ward of Bellevue Hospital. He was there for five days before his high fever was discovered, and he was transferred to another hospital for neurological workup. One aspect of this extremely traumatic episode was his embarrassment at having been in a psychiatric ward. He felt so humiliated that he did not tell his wife of many years; in fact, with his mother now dead, he alone knew. The doctor is urging him to tell his wife:

The-the fear involves the-the terror of-of-of the situation arising again and being misdiagnosed and nobody knowing what the past history was and then going through the same—

Tell your wife, will you?

Yeah.

Tell the whole story to your wife.

Yeah.

I'll tell you—

Yeah.

—examples of why. When I was in the service, we took care of what were called the Polish Guards. The Polish Guards were, were, uh—this was in France. I was stationed in France. The Polish Guards were Poles in the United States Army outside of, uh, you know, Communist Poland, right? So the guy comes in and he's— and he bumped his head. And he comes in and his eye was doing this— we call this, this motion, nystagmus, it's a very important diagnostic motion. We're saying, "Jesus, this guy must have a this and a that" and we're ready to go hnnnnn and the whole thing. He didn't speak any English. We don't speak any Polish. But there is just the possibility that every once in a while, uh, this motion is congenital. So, we're trying to find someone, another Polish Guard, who can speak enough English to talk to this guy before we go ship him off through the whole— right?

Right.

And, yeah, it was congenital.

So you're— you're inferring that what I had may be congenital and passed on to my—

No, I'm inferring that what you had was probably, uh, was probably encephalitis.

You probably did not think the physician was inferring that the patient's problem was congenital and that what he had might be "passed onto my ..." You probably guessed, correctly, that the doctor was giving a reason why someone else should know of his past history. The fears raised by that illness of many years earlier are still dictating the meaning he assigns to the doctor's words.

It is well known that people's perceptions are often guided by their own needs, desires, fears, and beliefs—conscious and unconscious; their perception of a speaker's intent may be similarly guided. A young woman came to see me because of pain in her sides that she was positive was due to damage to her ovaries from "sexual abuse," alone and in concert with others. After examining her, I told her that the pain had nothing to do with her ovaries and was muscular in origin. Because of her worries I went into the nature and treatment of her pain very carefully. While I was speaking to her, her eyes were shifted up and to the left, directed over my right shoulder. This is a sure sign that someone is not listening to you, but rather to some inner message. I finally said, "Rose, what did I just tell you?" She said "I must take care of myself, and I mustn't ..." I had said none of this. Finally, with some difficulty and with prompting, she remembered what I told her. Then I asked her what she would tell her mother I had advised. Once again, she said "He told me that I had to take care of myself ..." Sometimes, when patients do this I say, "You're listening with your fears, not with your ears." They are in fact supplying their own intent.

Requesting Confirmation
A second mechanism for reducing uncertainty is for speakers and hearers to test their interpretations, as the conversation progresses, by asking questions or asking the speaker to repeat a point. The speaker may say, "Right?" requesting confirmation. Often listeners do not question when they should, but in this next example the doctor is quite specific in testing whether the patient understood his question.

Are you having trouble concentrating on what you read at times?
Yeah, well, maybe it's eh, uh, the word, I don't know, but I read and I have to, to read again, to s— to see— what is it contains.
Are there times when you do not have to do that?
No, lately has been bad.

All the time? Every time you read?

About a year ago yes. From this—

No, you still don't understand me. Every time you read, now, do you have to reread?

When I read now, yes.

Each time?

Depending on the article or piece. A very, very simple, I— I get it easy.

Do you have any trouble with your handwriting?

No. No, but I haven't been writing too mu— too much.

Well, do you sign your name once in a while?

Yes, I sign—it and—

Is there . . . any change in your signature?

Oh, I think it is, it's so like, a— shaky?

Any trouble with your walking—balance?

Mm . . .

Do you feel weak in an arm or leg?

I've been feeling very weak, yes, one— one side that—

Now what is it that I just asked you?

If I feel weak when I— I've been feeling the loosing the balance when I walk.

No, I asked you if you feel weak in one arm—or one leg.

Oh, in one— In one leg, yes . . .

Which leg?

The left . . . It's weak. Always have been weak.

Since when?

Since—I was a little girl.

Why, did you have any— polio or anything?

No . . . No.

Any pain in the leg?

No.

Have you fainted at all? Do you see double?

No.

Any trouble swallow-ing? or Chewing?

No. No.

Any noise in the ear or deafness.

Uh, lately the ear bothers me . . .

The physician knows that, for whatever reason, he has an inattentive listener. He must ensure her comprehension of his questions. Not only do hearers use devices to test the intent of the speaker, but speakers also test and retest. This last point is particularly important to doctors, since it is essential that patients understand what they mean.

After saying to the patient, "Rather than the pills, one pill on two days, and the alternate pills on two days, three days on the third pill, and if you double pills up on the first day of each week after that, I think if you took one of those pills that you took last week, you'll have less trouble with the . . . if you're still taking those first pills," it would be reasonable to inquire whether the patient understood the directions. A direct, "Do you understand?" may not do the job, however, because some people believe that it is impolite to say "No." Instead, you can ask the patient to repeat the instructions to you. In so asking, the blame for failing to understand must be removed from the patient, so that it does not seem as though you think the patient is dumb. Instead, you can say "I'm not sure I made that very clear; could you please tell me what I just suggested?" or, "I apologize for asking, but this is very important: would you please repeat the medication instructions, so that I know I made myself clear." As the patient repeats the instructions, you may be awestruck at what you hear. You will know you are getting better at giving instructions, however, when your instructions start coming back to you the way you intended. As well as explaining verbally, I usually write things down. Once a patient brought back my written instructions a week later, saying, apologetically, that thay were incomprehensible. Indeed they were; I could not figure out what I meant. Naturally, it is crucial not only that you understand the patient but that the patient comprehend exactly what you mean, and you must check and recheck to make sure you have been understood. Knowing that pitfalls to understanding are present in the best of circumstances, and that sick, frightened, worried people have even more difficulty comprehending what may be essential information, you must spend time ensuring that the patient knows precisely what you do (and do not) mean. Spending such time is ultimately time saved, not wasted.

Redundancy
Another conversational mechanism that helps reduce uncertainty is redundancy. This is one of the most striking characteristics of the spoken language. Virtually every conversation is full of repetitions, rephrasings, simplifications, and explanations. Characteristically a speaker says something and then says it over and over again. Larded in among the repetitions are phrases such as, "Ya know what I

mean?" "D'ya know?" "Didja hear?" "Got me?" "Right?" and others, varying from region to region and dialect to dialect. This is why it is so difficult to produce a written paper from the transcript of an oral presentation. Every word in the written language can be read and reread to ensure understanding or check for errors of interpretation. Speech, however, is irreducibly linear, like time. Most listeners do not seem to remember what was literally said for more than a few moments, so that for ideas to remain current in the hearer's ears, the speaker must present them again and again. However, an attentive medical listener must learn to retain what was said in its literal form if the observation is to be separated from the interpretation.

Redundancy is even part of the written language. For example, every word in the phrase, "these three men," speaks of more than one: "these," rather than "that," telegraphs that the next word will describe something greater than one; "men," rather than "man," restates the fact. It is this redundancy intrinsic to syntax that allows one to guess the next word in a phrase with greater than random accuracy: after "these" and "three," the next word cannot be "man" or "boy." Redundancy decreases uncertainty and increases the probability that the listener will understand the speaker's intent. Since this is the desire of speakers in normal conversation, there should be signs in normal conversation that a listener can guess what is coming next. Ordinary conversation does in fact have considerable predictability. For example, if I say, "You know that old man who used to come to clinic every day? Well did you hear that he ..." you can probably supply the next word. Most listeners will say 'died." It could also have been "inherited a million dollars." But the phrase contains, "who used to come," implying that he no longer comes. And "Did you hear that he" implies that something happened. The words, "old man," contribute to the probability, as do the words "to clinic," and "everyday" suggests to us that he may have had a chronic illness. Thus built into the utterance is the expectation that when old men no longer come to clinic, it is more often because they died than because they met with good fortune.

You may argue that these indicators of the probability of the old man's death are not part of the language in the same manner as redundance is part of the grammar of "these three men." Such cues concern intent, and intent, as I pointed out in the beginning of the chapter, is characteristic of persons. Sentences and words cannot have intents; they can only have meanings. When a speaker wants to transmit meaning, he or she draws on a repertoire of words and phrases, knowledge of the social rules of conversation, knowledge of shared culture, self-knowledge, knowledge of context, and the history of interactions between speaker and listener. These are not, strictly speaking, part of language, but they are, without question, part of human communication. Our knowledge of how spoken communication works is primitive because these other aspects of understanding are more difficult to study than single words. Investigating artificial conversations in the laboratory has not led to deep understanding of spoken communication; yet the study of natural conversation has many difficulties, and little research has been carried out until quite recently.

I have tried to demonstrate that a listener's interpretation of what a speaker means is based on internal features within the utterances, on the context of speech, and on knowledge and expectations that both speaker and hearer bring to the conversation. Furthermore these interpretations can be tested against the constant repetition and redundancy that occurs in speech. When you become aware of these features, you can bring this knowledge to bear to interpret what people mean, test your interpretations, and make sure you are understood.

Reference

Byrne, Patrick S., and Barrie E. L. Long. *Doctors Talking to Patients*. London. Her Majesty's Printing Office, 1976, p. 136.

5

Words and Their Meanings

In chapter 2 I described the advantages of the world of language over the real world. Because of language we can act on the *word* for something rather than on the thing itself. Everyone, for example, has a body. The existence of the body is an objective fact. The notions of the body that are symbolized by the word "body," however, have certain advantages over the real thing, because language allows us to (figuratively) view it from different perspectives. We can make the body larger or smaller, stronger or weaker, bring it closer or distance it, all by changing the words used to describe it: the nouns, verbs, adverbs, adjectives, and pronouns with which the body or its parts will be associated in utterances. You may remember from chapter 2 the woman who distanced herself from her leg by saying, "My left leg is the bad leg from the vascular point of view. I had a thrombophlebitis in it," instead of, say, "I had thrombophlebitis in my left leg, my bad leg." This capacity of language is very functional, because it allows people to manipulate many parts of their world simply by changing the words they use. The same feature is also useful for physicians in their care of patients, because it allows the careful listener to learn about someone by noting the choice of words describing objects, events, and relationships. Physicians can also employ the capacity of language to manipulate reality by helping patients distance themselves, when necessary, from a disease or a diseased part: "I can't make that liver better, but I can help you."

In this chapter I am going to discuss a related dimension of language that makes it possible for words, signs, and symbols to play such a central role in human existence: the internal content of the notion signified by a word. This internal content consists of what a word *means* to a speaker. Philosophers call this the *intension* of the word, as opposed to the *extension*. The *extension* of the word "apple" is the fruit that grows on trees, and the *intension* is the content the speaker associates with the word "apple."

I want very much *not* to enter the interminable debate over the meaning of meaning. That scholars have spent so much time and energy trying to understand what follows from the statement "the word 'apple' means . . ." is a tribute to the complexity of the issue and the primitiveness of our understanding. Rather than joining the battle on the meaning of meaning, this book focuses specifically on how to use language in medicine. This chapter is designed to teach you how to use, in the service of the sick, the inner content in the minds of patients and doctors that is associated with words, signs, and symbols. If you wish to pursue the problem of meaning further, the bibliography contains the names of several books that will provide a good start. As this chapter proceeds, however, it will become clear why there has been so much debate about the meaning of words. As physicians we are fortunate to be able to ignore the philosophical debate, concentrating rather on the content that words evoke.

First, I will show some common traits of thought and indicate the way in which words fit into these thinking patterns. Then, I will show some of the things that can happen when a doctor attaches a name to a set of symptoms. I will then demonstrate that words not only activate thoughts and emotions, they can influence the body and have transcendant dimensions as well. Finally, I will indicate how all this fits in with the trained use of the spoken language in the care of patients.

A good place to start is with people's intense need to know the cause of events. Once, while teaching a course, I used hidden speakers to broadcast the sound of an adding machine. The volume was gradually turned up until the sound was distinct, but not loud enough to interfere with my speaking voice. The students turned this way and that, looking for the origin of the strange noise, apparently unable to put the sound out of mind so that they could concentrate on the lecture. So it is with all of us. Whenever anything occurs, we are driven to know its origin or cause. Illness is such an occurrence. Note these next two examples:

Now, if they kill the antibio— the antibodies that are creating the platelet loss, what does that mean?
Well, we're hoping—
Does that mean that you've found—
We're hoping that the antibodies— We're hoping—
—That you've found— found the cause, or—

We're hoping that—I will only discuss it briefly. First I want to make a categorical statement. You did NOT cause your own multiple sclerosis.
I don't believe you!
That's all right.

These were two sick people who, like all patients, want to know the cause of their illness. If questions about cause are not raised directly, they show up in some other manner. In seeking the cause of their illness, most people develop some interesting notions about why it occurred. It may not surprise you to find out that many patients believe that something about themselves caused their illness: something they did or did not do, ate or did not eat, thought or did not think. These notions may be believed despite overwhelming evidence to the contrary. The phenomenon is so ubiquitous as to be almost invisible.

Here is another brief example.

You going to ask me anything else so that we make sure we know all about everything?
Um, if the person has an enlarged liver. Is there a majority of why—in other words, eighty percent could be this and ten percent could be that, or ninety percent could be this and five percent could be that?

As I have suggested, the search for cause is not only present among the sick. Suppose that one evening you leave home, locking things securely in your usual fashion. On returning, you find two chairs in the living room not in their usual position and not, you are certain, the way you left them. A search of the rooms reveals nothing else missing or disturbed. Most people, in such circumstances, will be very worried and unable to put the matter from their minds. Occurrences like this are used in mystery movies to set the stage for the strange events to follow, since the audience knows that something or somebody must have moved those chairs! We all know that every event must have a cause.

I believe that the need to determine the cause of things is part of the way we deal with uncertainty. Understanding the importance of reducing uncertainty may clarify why people always seek to explain events. Once an occurrence has been assigned a cause, the uncertainty produced by the event (What is it? What should I do about it?) subsides. Until then *the matter cannot be put out of mind.* Hence, in the example I cited, the class could not pay attention to the lecture and kept searching for the origin of the hidden sound even though the actual noise volume did not interfere with hearing the lecture.

Stigmatized individuals—patients with obvious deformities or disabilities, the ugly, the obviously ill, those who are different from most others in a group—also "require an explanation." It is as though the order of one's internal world must be maintained by finding reasons for any change from the usual. When my daughter was six, she played with a friend whose mother had cerebral palsy. On returning home the first time, she said, referring to the mother, "It's hard not to stare at her." Staring was apparently the natural thing to do when the child saw a person who looked different from anyone else she had ever seen. Her notions about persons, what they look like and how they behave, were briefly destabilized, to be put in order again by "that's because she has cerebral palsy, darling." In describing this, I am expanding the concept of uncertainty, suggesting that uncertainty comes about whenever a person confronts something—an object, event, or relationship—that does not "fit" the person's notions about the world. Rather than change beliefs, it is easier to "find a cause," to seek out a reason consistent with previous ideas. The whole structure of beliefs then remains intact. When phrased this way, physicians may recognize a biological principle with which we have long experience: homeostasis, the maintenance of the status quo. Just as the cellular milieu is defended against change, so too is the person's structure of beliefs.

Why is this important to the care of patients? It is essential for doctors to realize that the same processes—searching for cause, attempting to reduce uncertainty, and defending the set of beliefs about the world against sudden change—are occurring at all times in their patients. These beliefs are tied to language. When individuals deal with happenings in their world, they work primarily on their internalized notions and the words that represent these notions, *not on reality itself.* Thus it is vitally important to understand all the dimensions of words and how they function, for it is through spoken words that the physician is able to influence the patient's reality.

To suggest that individuals deal primarily with representations of reality—words—rather than with reality itself does not seem to do justice to the immediacy of personal experience: the moment-by-moment living of life with all its happenings and perceived sensations. In fact experience and words interact: word meanings are adapted and changed to conform with reality, and words can help "alter" reality to conform with the individual's meaning system.

We can imagine a process, with words and their meanings at one end and "booming, buzzing confusion" at the other. Normally, despite individual differences of detail, there is a "semantic baseline" made up of meanings shared by all language users. Language holds society together; we would all become unstuck if, due to completely ideosyncratic meanings, we were unable to communicate, and so one aspect of the reality to which an individual's meanings must adapt are the meanings of others. This does not imply that people cannot have idiosyncratic word meanings. It does suggest, however, that *some* of the notions attached to each word must be common to the community of speakers. In other words, people can share some of their meanings with many and some with few others. Every husband or wife has experience with meanings that are private between the two of them. In psychosis, the process is shifted, so that there is little adaptation of individual meanings to conventional usage; since such conventions are the basis for a common reality, the psychotic is, literally, "in another world."

Note the following examples, as we explore these concepts:

Two weeks ago, I'm sitting in my office and I start getting these spots in front of my eyes. I couldn't see anything. I was— you know, nothing. I was just—seeing these little, crazy little spots. Which I've had that before, but maybe for a minute, or not even a minute. A couple of seconds or something, I'll see spots.

So I said, "Well, you know, I'll stand up, I'll walk around, it'll go away. I'll take out my lenses." I figured, "It's the lens—." I wear soft lenses. So I popped out the soft lenses, and the spots didn't go away so I took a walk and I got as far as the Art Department and I couldn't— well, for one thing I was blind without my lenses and I'm sort of walking like this.

But really it wasn't just the spots, it was a combination of things. At that point I didn't really have a headache, I don't think, I just felt slightly dizzy or something. It was a couple of weeks ago, I don't remember exactly. But I sat down in there and I was figuring, "Well, what is this?" And I started getting these shooting pains in this side. It was just like all— everywhere. And it just made me a little bit upset. I figured, "Well, didn't have anything to eat too much this morning. I'll go across the street to the Beanery, you know, and get something to eat."

So I got up from the Art Department and I went down and I was standing on the corner of 52nd Street and Madison Avenue and all of a sudden I just— I guess 'cause I was worried because nothing like this really, I don't think, ever happened to me—well, I know it didn't—shooting pains in my head and because I was scared about that, I think this is why this happened, but I felt compelled to hold on to a tel— a metal pole thing, like this, 'cause I started feeling woozy.

And then I figured, "Ah, I'm going to get into that place and have some orange juice, and high protein stuff, I'll feel better."

Then the light changed and I jus— I don't know what happened. Just sort of, my knees went out from under me. I just fell down and I was carrying my coat, and my coat dropped, so I just went down like this, I got my coat, and I stood up, you know, so that it (I guess) looked to people like I dropped my coat and I just— you know. But really that isn't what happened. I fell down first.

I go into the place and I say to the guy, "Give me this, this, and this." And I ordered some stuff and I'm waiting for it— No, I'm sitting there and th-th— it's sort of getting kind of worse and all of a sudden— I just get— and then I— I'm— I'm trying to keep sort of in touch. Like I'm saying, "Well, this is all psychosomatic, or something like that. Nothing bad is going to happen." And then I just sort of freaked out just for a little tiny bit and I just had this horrible image— I had this image that my brains were like bleeding or something. It was very strange. And I just figured, like, "Ah! This is curtains. I'm going to croak. I'm not going to get out of this place!" And I kept thinking, "Isn't it funny how, I'm sure that people must die of embarrassment. Because I'm in a drugstore. I could have gone—if I was really that scared, I thought I was going to die. I figured, "This must be a hemorrhage or something," and started thinking of all these things. But I didn't want to bother the guy in the back to say, "Well, call my doctor," or something.

And then what happened a little bit after that is-is that I got this headache, like a regular headache, like right in the front, like I've had before and it was terrible. But I took some aspirins and stuff, but I was— because I can deal with that. I knew what that was. And then it wasn't until I was OK , I guess. The headache finally went away. It took a couple of hours but the other thing was fine. And I told a friend about this and she said, "Oh! Well, for Christ sake, that was a migraine!" And I thought— I said, "Ah!" (Snap) I mean I didn't— if I had thought of it when it happened, I probably would have felt much better.

Happiness is a word called "migraine." The patient is more articulate than most, but what she relates is well known to all of us. Migraine is not a cause, it is a word. Why then does it function for this woman as a cause? If it had occurred to her that she was having a migraine headache, then all the frightening things that happened would have been explained. No uncertainty would have existed, into which terrifying possibilities might intrude. You may disagree, suggesting that migraine can cause all the symptoms the woman manifested. I think not. "Migraine" is merely a name, a label that physicians have assigned to a cluster of phenomena—symptoms and signs—that may occur in patients. The cause of these symptoms is not "migraine"; "migraine" *stands for* those symptoms. The cause in fact is unknown.

Confusion between the word for something and the thing itself is extraordinarily common. One type of confusion, of particular concern to physicians, is *reification*: the error of misplaced concreteness. Thus the word "migraine" gives a solidity to the series of phenomena for which it is the label, that sneaks it into the class of well-defined clinical entities. The phenomenon itself, however, is *not* (yet) well defined. As a somewhat banal example, take the word "hypoglycemia," used as a diagnosis (usually by laypersons). The symptoms of nervousness, sweatiness, weakness, and various other discomforts, which most laypersons mean to suggest when they use the word, take place as the blood sugar drops rapidly below a certain point. They may follow the sympathetic response that occurs with the fall in blood sugar. The symptoms are only one manifestation of the whole chain of events involved in the regulation of blood glucose. The word "hypoglycemia," when used as a label, is very much more concrete and coherent than the disordered process of blood sugar control to which it is often applied. When, to that confusion, one adds the fact that the label "hypoglycemia" is perhaps most often used when no abnormalities of blood sugar control are demonstrable, then the problem of believing something to be a concrete entity because there exists a word for it is more easily grasped.

In this next example the patient uses words in much the same way.

And then the other thing connected with it, as I realize now in retrospect only, for about three weeks I've been doing this all the time: stretching, as if I had a pulled muscle or something. And I go to exercise class once a week and I noticed when I bend the leg I felt weak on that side but I really didn't pay any attention to it. 'Cause sometimes you get a pulled—something. And suddenly it began to hurt horribly and I realized it was my kidney! It wasn't my back at all! And it hurt very badly.

What made you realize that it was your kidney?

An acute pain here.

Mm-hm. How do you connect it?

I connect it with Sansert. Now I may be absolutely wrong, but it's the only—

How long have you been on the Sansert?

About two years. A year and a half, two years.

Now, how do you connect the knees, ankles, and your kidneys?

Only if it has to do with water somewhere. I mean, it's completely amateur commonsense analysis, but something's being retained somewhere. I don't know why, I shouldn't even presume to answer that. I don't know the answer. Only that Goodgold did tell me something I remembered.

I don't care what he said.

Yeah, but.... He read me the textbook thing.

Mm-hm.

The contraindications and all that and he said the only real danger—the reason you have urinalysis, is there is potential damage to the kidneys.

Right, now—

And that suddenly came back to me—

Up until—I'm not counting these three events: ankles, knees, and kidneys—up until this week, have you been feeling well?

Yes. And let me tell you, the Sansert works. When I go off it—that's a funny thing because I had THAT for many years and it was never diagnosed. Chuck said I had electroencephalograms and I had what I call "the Bette Davis test," the "Dark Victory" test. I was grand. There was nothing wrong with me. And Chuck kept saying, "Well, it's one of those things—" you know how he is. "Leave me alone." Except that every three weeks it got worse and worse and worse, and it's completely frightening because you have vertigo, double vision—it's very frightening. Finally, he found Goodgold somewhere—newly on the horizon, and he sent me to see him, and he diagnosed it as "migraine equivalent" and said I shouldn't have it any more at my age but I do.

Have you ever had any trouble with your kidneys?

Never. I've always had superb kidneys.

There were remarkably few symptoms in that recitation. If one really wanted to know what happened, it would take considerable questioning to find out what those words meant to her. This phenomenon, of a patient reciting a series of diagnoses instead of symptoms, occurs frequently. "When I had my ulcer, which was the same time my sinusitis turned into bronchitis . . ." For those patients, providing the name of something somehow takes the place of telling about the thing.

Diagnoses—the names given to afflictions—have many functions. The diagnosis can serve the function of reducing uncertainty, of moving the events from the unknown to the known. The diagnostic label serves to contain the threat. Sometimes, as we shall see, the diagnosis mitigates the threat because of the information it conveys about cause, course, and outcome. This, however, is not always the case. Much medical humor comes from the lack of content of some medical terms. A man has a painful tailbone and is satisfied to be told that his trouble is coccyalgia or coccydynia—both of which merely mean painful tailbone. The power is in the name.

As a resident at Bellevue I had a patient who was persistently dissatisfied with our lengthy explanations of his condition. My intern satisfied him by saying that his problem was a "gastric stomach." Why was the patient then content? The "diagnosis" did not reveal cause, characteristics, and outcome. The humor (for the intern) derived from the fact that the patient was happy knowing he had a "stomach" stomach. If he were aware that to have a gastric stomach was simply to have a stomach stomach, he would have been insulted, not satisfied. What function, then, did the name serve for that patient? For one thing, he believed that his physician knew the name of his disease, and thus knew all that is implied in the conception for which the name is the label. If the doctor knows, than the patient is provided the same comfort that comes from knowing, himself. But more, the very fact of a name signifies that the thing is known. Labeling in itself indicates the move from unknown to known, providing the comfort and reduction in uncertainty that goes with a known object. Further the label, or signifier, can then be manipulated as though the object itself were being manipulated. Moreover the fact that physicians can name something may imply that they can do something. To name the beasts of the field implies the power to dominate them.

In addition patients wish to know the name of their illness for social reasons. They have to tell their families and and friends why they are in the hospital. Not to be able to answer the inevitable questions by providing the diagnosis, casts doubt on the quality of medical care and the competence of one's physicians. The absence of a name allows worry to seek its own name. If the patient's family were able only to recite the symptoms, saying that the doctors did not know what was wrong, their listeners would have doubts. The listeners would wonder whether someone was avoiding the whole truth and, in not telling the name, concealing a more terrible truth. Newspaper obituaries often read, "He died after a long illness," instead of "He died from cancer." If the facts are being concealed, the listeners may wonder who is avoiding the truth—the patient, the family, the doctors? Consider how dependent interpersonal relationships are on the sharing of knowledge and how much meaning is read into the absence of a name. Patients need to know the name of their disease so that they can justify their absence from work and their relief from other obligations.

The name is the public justification for the assumption of the sick role. Aside from its technical aspects, the name is useful for doctors, serving as a vehicle for corridor and coatroom conversation. It also serves as a shorthand that allows physicians to share their burdens with one another without being explicit about their concerns: "I just admitted a lady with late stage ALM" (amyotrophic lateral sclerosis). "Too bad. That's a drag." All the problems connected with the care of patients with advanced muscle disease are well known to physicians; that brief interchange acknowledges the doctor's difficulties without the necessity of speaking about feelings, as well as many other issues that would be complex at best, and inexplicable at worst. The use of jargon, such as "ALM," is, in itself one of the communal functions of symbols. Patients with the same disease sometimes forge a community of sufferers in which part of the right to belong is familiarity with the in-group language. All of these functions, and more, are served by the diagnosis. "I heard you were in the hospital lately." "Yes." "What was the matter?" "I had diverticulitis." "Oh! You had diverticulitis … I had an uncle who had diverticulitis. I know he had a lot of trouble. Were you very sick?" (Etc.) The label diverticulitis is very functional for people. They have uncles who have it. Diverticulitis is something that will keep you out of work for X amount of time. Diverticulitis is not cancer, but on the other hand, you are not faking. This interaction operates through the symbol "diverticulitis."

I would surmise that diverticulitis has a meaning in all those statements that differs from its meaning when used by physicians. The name of the disease—the symbol that stands for what is happening to the patient—may have a very different content in order to serve its various functions. For doctors it has one meaning; for the patient, another; for the family, yet another—but rarely in such situations are people aware of all of the internal content of the conception for which the name stands. Some of the notions could be called to awareness if someone probed for them, but other parts of the conception remain below awareness.

In these next examples I probed to find out what name the patients had attached to their symptoms. In each instance the disease that came to mind was serious; indeed, that is almost always the case. The examples were taped in 1969, when I was first exploring the beliefs that patients had about their symptoms. I am sure, however, that you can confirm these findings this year, and perhaps a hundred years from now (although the names will change), because for the patient, and others, finding a name is essential.

What do you think this is all due to?
I don't know—
Well, when you're thinking about your insides, what do you think it is?
I don't know—
Well you must have some kind of—
A disease—or some kind of—
What kind of disease?
Well that's what I want to find out—
Yeah, but what do you think? I mean, everybody has some ideas.
Well, you know maybe it's cancer of the stomach or maybe it's nerves, or an ulcer. An ulcer. That's what I think it might be. An ulcer.
Is that bad?
Yeah!
Why.
An ulcer? That's ridiculous! For a woman to get an ulcer.
Why?
Well it shows that you have all this tension within you.

What do you think this is?
I don't know, Doctor.
Well, everybody thinks about their health, so what do you put it together as?
Well, I had some crazy idea that maybe I had a cancer of some kind, of— (laughter) the stomach or colon, I mean I—
What are the other possibilities besides the cancer of the stomach?
I can't think of any.

What do you think it is?
I have no idea. I don't know if it's my back, I don't know why I have the pains in my legs and my arms, unless it's a pinched nerve—
Mm-hm. When you're worried about it, what do you think it is?
When I get carried away, I think a brain tumor or something!

Why does each one find a name, and why is the disease always serious? I can only speculate that even a bad disease is better than total uncertainty, and that a serious interpretation of symptoms may help spur the patient to take action. When patients do not come up with a name, they may have a sense of dread: a foreboding of "terrible" and "horrible," to which no name is attached. When pushed, however, they do not say "terrible" or "horrible"; they accept names like "cancer" or "multiple sclerosis." This next example illustrates the point that a name, however serious its implications, can reduce uncertainty.

Well, cancer's what bothers me.

You mean the possibility that that's there?

Right.

I don't know it to be true. Was that the first time that it crossed your mind?

What do you mean?

It hadn't crossed your mind before that?

No, because I'm not familiar with that type—

You mean in all the time you had been ill it had never crossed your mind?

No. But that's not a popular type.

Mm-hm. What isn't a popular type?

The lymph— lymph nodes or something. Lymph nodes?

What lymph nodes? Where did you get lymph nodes? I didn't say anything about lymph nodes—

No?

No. Who said that? Well you better tell me— You mean what all that feeling was for?

Yeah.

Nothing.

Oh. I thought I had lymph nodes or something.

No. No. No. No, no. In fact, that was my polite way of telling Dr.——, the intern who saw you, that I thought it was nothing, without in front of you saying, "I think that's nothing."—No. I didn't— who's told you you had cancer of the lymph nodes? I didn't tell you that— What did I tell you yesterday? If you have a question, to ask me?

Mm-hm. But lymph nodes was mentioned at the time. And I got the impression that the two were related.

Didn't I tell you yesterday specifically, "Don't be in such a rush to get into trouble. You'll get there on time"

The patient had metastatic carcinoma to the liver from the bowel and was being examined for lymphadenopathy which had been reported by another physician. She asked what was being done and was told that the doctors were feeling for enlarged lymph nodes. Then, without further explanation, they departed. Behind them they left the words "lymph nodes" which, lacking other explanation, she put together with cancer.

"Rose Is a Rose, Is a Rose, Is a Rose."

I have been suggesting, throughout this chapter, that for each symbol, whether word or image, the person has a conception. "Conception" is more appropriate here than "concept," because conception implies the process of conceiving a notion or an idea, something always in flux, whereas concept implies a more static and fixed entity. Symbols and their meanings do change over time, and therefore the more active word is preferred.

In these next examples we see some of the content of the conceptions people hold. What we are reading is what these patients had in mind when they talked about certain issues. Incidentally, note that some of the signs are complex: not a single word, but several. In this next example, the noun is not "fluid," but rather "fluid-in-the-abdomen." One often hears jokes about German compound nouns made up of several words. We do the same in English, however, conceptually if not lexically.

Because, something's causing it, isn't it?
Yes, something's causing it. Is that a surprise to you? That you got fluid in your belly?
No, it just frightens me, that's all.
Well, what frightens you about it? What's frightening about it?
Well, I feel each time it fills up you gotta empty it.
Well, is it the emptying that's frightening?
Yeah.
You mean the actual physical doing of it that's frightening.
And then testing the, ah—
So the fear is that somebody'll do that and find cancer cells in it?
Yeah.
Listen, . . . , that fluid is probably related to that cancer, it just doesn't have to have cells from it. And you don't care about that you care about what it's doing to you.
Right.
And if you're going to look at that as though there's some big, you know, accumulation of cancer and that's what that swelling is—
No, I don't think I've ever looked at it like that—

The "fluid-in-the-abdomen" is conceived of as having cancer cells. You may wonder whether the notion occupying her is "fluid-in-the-abdomen" or "cancer," since the two seem to interact in the utterance. The reason that it is sometimes difficult to tell which conception is at issue will become clearer as we proceed. Note this next example.

I have a vaginal infection that I've had for three months.
Three months?
Yes. I have been to a doctor three times and I've been treated with Penicillin and, you know, stuff you put up in you, and for a yeast infection, and it has not helped it go away. And I'm getting very perturbed.
Now, have you ever had a vaginal infection like this before?
I've had infections before, but they always went away. I had it when I was married. But then it would always clear up. So I never had one that just went on and on and on. I thought maybe some of my pneumonia virus snuck down there (laughter) and— I don't know.

"Vaginal-infections," which she has had before, always go away. Is this a "vaginal-infection" like the others, or is it different—perhaps a "pneumonia-virus-vaginal-infection." Or is the utterance not about "vaginal-infection" as much as it is about various infections, such as "yeast-infection" (which always went away with antibiotics) versus "pneumonia-virus-infection" (against which antibiotics would be ineffective)? With the evidence given we can only speculate, but the example hints at the complexity of the notions related to the words a speaker employs.

In this next example some of the content of the conception "prednisone" is given by another person who accompanies the patient. Note that the words "cortisone" and "prednisone" are used interchangeably.

So there should be no confusion, unless I SPECIFICALLY TELL YOU, "*Stop the prednisone.*"
Mm-hm.
Prednisone is always tapered off.
(Friend) Her face will get rou— Your face will get round, but don't get excited. Doesn't it?
What?
(Friend) From the cortisone.
No.
(Friend) No it will not?
No. You'll have no side effects at this—
But it starts to jus—

No. Not like that, no.
(Friend) No?
No. Not like that.
(Friend) Just a little.
No!
(Friend) Not at all?
Not at all.
(Friend) Very good.

In this next example the conception "prostate" is at issue.

The problem with the prostrate is it's just a frustrating thing. There's not much you can do about it.
Well, why— what does it make you think is going to happen?
That I'll eventually have to have it removed.
Well, suppose you had your prostate taken out. What would that mean to you? When you think about it, what is it you think about?
Well, the prostrate, from what I know, supplies the fluid to get the sperm moving into the— the cervix.
Well, when people don't have their prostate removed, they really don't have that prostate removed. They just have the benign tumor that's on top of the prostate removed. They still have a prostate.
And it still furnishes the fluid for— having sex?
You mean, if you didn't have that fluid you wouldn't have sex?
No, it could be that you wouldn't be able to have children in a normal way.
In other words, you'd be impotent.
Possibly.
So is the fear of sterility or impotence?
Mostly sterility.

This example demonstrates an extremely common set of misconceptions about prostatic disease. I once saw a patient whose notions about the prostate and prostatectomy led to a self-fulfilling prophecy. When asked why he stopped having intercourse, became obese, and appeared eunachoid, he said that he knew those things happened after a prostatectomy. Although, because of retrograde ejaculation after transurethral prostatectomy, no ejaculate will be visible, none of those beliefs are true. Because the patient believed them, however, they came to pass. The same phenomenon can be observed in women who have had a hysterectomy and who believe the dire mythology about the deterioration that is said by some to follow the operation. The point is that the content of a conception is like a set of operating instructions which the person must either follow or alter. I pointed out earlier that it is often simpler to change reality than one's beliefs. As we shall see below, the interconnectedness of conceptions makes it difficult for persons to change one set of ideas without changing their whole structure of beliefs.

Every physician has heard something like this next example:

I can drink water?

Sure.

I love to drink water. I've been dying to drink water.

Drink all you want.

Ok. Ok. 'Cause I was afraid to drink it when I was home because my ankles swelled up.

Mm-hm.

What was the cause of my ankles swelling up?

Your liver is pressing on the big vein that comes from the legs and just makes them—water has nothing to do with that. You don't retain water because you drank it. And if you don't drink water, you'll get yourself sick.

I see. I tried to stay away from all liquids so that my ankles wouldn't swell.

No.

What she said seems to make sense. If there is fluid retention in the ankles it must be because one takes in too much fluid. When you explain that the primary problem is the retention of salt, not water, the patient may not believe you and a lengthy explanation may be required. Too frequently physicians act very superior in these situations because of the patients' ignorance. Everyone, however, no matter how knowledgeable, holds some silly beliefs. In a series of interviews I once conducted about why patients developed infectious diseases, relatively sophisticated young physicians could be pushed to the point where they revealed that they believed that the patient may have done something "bad" (in the moral sense), and that this was the cause of the illness.

Sometimes the content of the patient's conception is so odd that you cannot conceive of its origin. Psychoanalytic theory has made this point for many years. This next example comes from a telephone conversation between myself and a woman with end-stage carcinoma of the lung. She had recurrent pleural effusions that were the source of most of her symptoms. One of her initial problems, solved by changing her conception of pleural effusion, was her belief that if her pleura filled up sufficiently she would die a horrible death because the fluid would spill over and she would drown. This example is a segment of a later conversation.

Look, Eric, one minute I think, "Look, I won't see this fall again. I'm going to die." And I accept it. And then the next day I don't accept it. And I don't panic. And I don't want to die.

That's reasonable, isn't it?

And I cry. I cry a great deal. And then I have had quite a little bit more pain than I've had before and in different areas. Oh. There was another question that a friend of mine asked me to ask Dr. H——; if every time they took— I've just been drawn. That's why I'm breathing nicely. I was drawn about three days ago. About a quart and a half, same amount. Do they test the junk that comes out? Well, H——said, "No, we throw it down the sink." Which they did, right in front of me.

Sure.

Well, because there's no point in— I guess they gather that the whole thing is swarming with spermatozoa cancer cells and—that's that!

Funny image.

Well, it's not so damn funny.

I mean, "spermatozoa cancer"—

No, but you see I associate spermatozoa with my cerebral palsy brother marrying his—I just hate the idea of sex, you see.

Mm-hm.

And all this is tied up with— spermatozoa to me is a horrid thing. And it's associated with cancer cells.

I have shown that people always try to find the cause of events and that, as with the lady and the migraine, merely pinning a name on something may do the job. Further the name of an illness serves many other functions as well. The preceeding examples demonstrate how much additional information may be associated with a symbol. Indeed, the symbol seems to be more like an information container than anything else.

Let me go further. In chapter 2 I pointed out the conventional wisdom that a conception is like a definition. It has a noun phrase, as in "*melanoma*: a malignant tumor whose parenchyma is composed of melanocytes." This is called the denotative definition. But when people speak about melanoma they add value judgments. It is a vicious tumor, or bad, nasty, dangerous. The words, as used, are usually containers of more than a denotative definition; they also include how speakers feel about the thing. This larger usage is called the connotative definition. Because most words, as used, have associated adjectives or adverbs that describe how the speaker feels about them, the everyday distinction between thinking and feeling does not hold up.

The examples in this chapter suggest that conceptions contain more than merely facts, as in the denotative definition, and more than facts plus values added by adjectives and adverbs. Conceptions also include information about where the thing for which the word stands comes from and what becomes of it. Everything seems to arise from something and go on to something else. Apples come from apple trees, and they become applesauce, or keep doctors away, or taste crunchy in the mouth, or become brown in spots. Malignant melanoma is not only a tumor whose parenchyma is composed of melanocytes, and not only vicious or dangerous; it comes from the transformation of certain cells, and it grows, spreads, and kills. Now we understand why the patient appeared relieved when she could say, "Oh it's a migraine." Migraines, common wisdom has it, come from "nerves" and from being a perfectionist; they never kill you or make your brains bleed. The conception, for which the word migraine is the sign, contains all this information and much more.

On a moment's reflection you will see that it would be almost impossible to have a conception isolated from all other conceptions. To use the word "migraine" implies knowledge about other headaches. The word "headache" also evokes content, some of which is the same as "migraine" and some different. But the two are related. And headache has the word "head," which evokes a different conception, and the word "pain," which is related to still others. A network of relationships between conceptions must exist, and this network is the whole structure of beliefs about the world held by an individual. When, as physicians, we talk to a patient, we are speaking to the person's conceptions. When you say "You are going to get prednisone," you may spark a whole chain of conceptual events—fears, worries, ideas, and action—for which you are unprepared, because you spoke from *your* conceptions but not, in addition, purposefully to *their* conceptions. If, however, we can change someone's conception by what we do or say, think of the potential for action this creates.

What has been presented thus far demonstrates many of the facets of language and the events that a word sets off. People, however, are more complex and their inner life more rich than has been exemplified thus far. Let us go on to explore more deeply the meaning of words and the functions of symbols.

The following examples come from hypnotized patients. For those readers with little or no experience with hypnosis let me explain the procedure that led to these interactions. A hypnotic trance was induced in which general relaxation was suggested. In the hypnotized state persons can have an awareness of, or produce physical sensations, emotional states, intellectual processes, and internal states not accessible to ordinary consciousness. Except for an occasional highly trained or disciplined person, the achievement of these phenomena requires the help of another, the hypnotist or operator, although the capacity resides in the subject. Thus to an individual in such a trance the operator can say, "You will feel sad," and the subject will feel sad; or, "You will begin to have the feeling in your body that just precedes your asthma attack," and the patient's throat will itch, their chest will tighten, they will cough, or experience whatever sensation is usual for them will occur. I must add that if the subject does not want this to occur, it will not. People do not do things they do not wish to do in a trance, although a situation can sometimes be suggested in which the subject finds something acceptable that would otherwise be offensive. No asthmatic wants to have asthma. But if it is suggested that by having an attack of asthma in a trance, they can learn to control their breathing better at other times, then patients may permit the asthma to happen.

These next examples are responses to the following suggestion: "You are going to have the feeling that goes with the words *I am.* Your whole body will be occupied by the feeling that goes with the words *I am!*

Mmm— it's splendid.

Describe it.

Well, first of all, I can feel— not the intellectual feelings— but the feelings are that I am completely from head to toe, I can feel there's an absolute connection there. And I feel that it's so relaxed, or something that if I got up, there might not even be any Joyce there. But I know it'll be OK because if I do get up, it'll work out and if I don't, it's very nice. And I also feel— I feel very big.

It's comfortable.

What does it feel like?

It feels like—it's really hard to describe. It doesn't feel like I'm floating, it just feels like I'm just in this chair and it's so comfortable.
What does your body feel like?
It feels good! It feels—it feels like it's sort of resting.
Mm-hm. Is it a weak feeling?
No.
Is it a restless feeling?
No.
Is it a content feeling?
Yeah. Very content.

Ohhh— That feels very good.
Mm-hm. What does it feel like? Describe it. Somewhat.
Oh it feels secure. It feels also protected. And protecting—

In this next, we see that "I am" is not necessarily pleasant:

My stomach's getting tight, I don't know—

One patient, who had had asthma since infancy, began to wheeze when asked to have the feeling that goes with "I am," as though asthma had become part of her identity or self-conception. This suggests the possibility that a physician wanting to make her asthma disappear would have threatened her identity!

One can also have feelings that go with the words "I want."

My body feels sort of tingly—
Unpleasant feeling?
Nm-mm.
Strong feeling?
Yeah!
Different from the "I am" feeling?
Yeah.
Mm-hm.

I can't— In a way, I don't feel the elation that I felt a moment ago, but I can't— It doesn't feel bad, and it doesn't feel—great.

What does it feel like?
Well, it doesn't feel great, just like a second ago.
What does THIS feeling feel like.
This just feels like— nice, but it doesn't have the dramatic feeling like "I am" feels like. It feels like I'm— I feel like I'm part of the chair and I'm relaxed in that sense. And I feel that every part of me is supported in a nice, sort of secure, way. I didn't get any other sort of, grand feelings from it.
Do you want to go back to "I am"? Go on back to "I am."

One further example:

What does that feel like?
I don't know—
Is it the same as the previous feeling? Is it the same as "I am"? "*I want,*" *is what this feels like.*
I want—
Is it a nice feeling?
Yeah—
Is it a strong feeling, or a weak feeling? A weak feeling or a small feeling?
I guess— I'm not too comfortable. I don't know what this—
It's not as comfortable, hm?
No.
Is your face tight?
Yeah. 'Cause—
Is your head tight?
Yeah. My head started getting tight when I started thinking about "I want." I don't know what I want—!

The point of all of these examples is that saying words like "I am" or "I want" causes these listeners to have body sensations. Subjects have also responded to "I want" with, "Wow, that feels great," or "Oh no, no, no, thats a no, no," while others have noted sexual feelings.

Once again, one might ask what this has to do with medicine. A young woman with asthma since childhood married a man with a dog. Not surprisingly, she developed attacks of asthma when the dog was present. This caused marital conflict. The husband accused his wife of having "psychological" attacks of asthma, because every time they had an argument about the dog, which he wanted to keep, she would start wheezing. When she was hypnotized, during an unrelated conversation, I suddenly said "Dog!"—and she started wheezing. By simply saying a word to that patient, I caused her to have acute airway obstruction! When this occurs, meaning has bridged the gap between the classic medical categories of subjective and objective. The wheezing that is caused is very real and is not merely shortness of breath; it is as real as the changes in the blood gases that take place.

Physicians sometimes have difficulty accepting the asthma induced in a trance as "real" asthma—as though it is perhaps different from the airway obstruction following exposure to allergens or cold air. It is true that a patient whose asthma has gone on for days will be different from one whose asthma was just started in a trance. But unfortunate personal experience has demonstrated to me that an asthma attack can be initiated in a hypnotized patient that will take hours and intravenous medication to terminate. One way of understanding this issue is to realize that the body as well as the mind is an information processor. Allergens carry information that is "read" by mast cells, air temperature is information to which twitchy airways react, the inspired air may contain irritants which carry information to which the airways also react. The flow of information to and from the body and its parts is characteristic of all living systems from cells to nations. One source of information to the body to which it may respond is carried by words. The only problem for most readers with what I am saying is a habit of thinking that has traditionally separated the mind (to which words belong) from the body. Thinking of mind and body as absolutely separate is an atavistic mode of thought that is difficult to part with precisely because of what is described in this chapter— the intertwined structure of beliefs, where changing one (central) notion requires change in so many other ideas.

It should be no surprise that, besides stimulating thoughts, words can cause things to happen in the body. All persons have heard utterances that made them "sick to the stomach" or gave them a chill or panicky physical feeling. But let me demonstrate the matter more systematically. In each of the following examples the hypnotized subject was told, by way of instruction, something like this: "I am talking as if there are different 'channels' into which a word can go when you hear it. For example, one such 'channel' is the thinking, cognitive mind. Another is the channel of affect—emotional feelings. A third is the somatic channel—physical feelings." (There is, in fact, a fourth "channel," but just as I did not tell the subjects about it in advance, I would prefer to delay telling you.)

This next patient is a thirty-seven-year-old psychologist being treated for carcinoma of the stomach. He had a subtotal gastrectomy after he perforated through a malignant ulcer. At the time of this interaction, many months later, he was receiving chemotherapy. The patient was in a trance.

You are going to get the feelings in your body that go with the word "mountains." Your body will fill with the feelings that go with the word "mountains." What does that feel like?

It's a very liberating feeling. It's a—to begin with, it's like—well, it's a meadow. And it's green and it has sun, and you feel good in walking and . . .

What does your BODY feel like?

In touch with itself. I mean, ah—

Are there feelings in your body that go with the word "mountain"?

Yeah. It's hard and soft at the same time. . . . . It's very strong, you know that?

Later in the same conversation the following exchange took place:

All right. You are going to get the sensations in your body and ONLY your body, the sensations that go with the word "chemotherapy."

It's pain.

Where? Do you have it now?

It's—

What do you sense now?

Nausea, and— nausea. And— a feeling of awkward— I mean, not awk— yeah, awkward—like I could vomit.

You are going to get the thoughts—

Revulsion. Revulsion.

Revulsion?

I don't know. I feel atrociously— not atrociously, but very badly nauseated.

You feel nauseated, do you?

Yes.

Very badly nauseated?

Yes.

Very badly nauseated?

Not that bad, but I mean—

Not good.

No.

And, further:

You are going to get the thoughts, and ONLY the channel of thoughts, do you understand? Only that channel. Now, thoughts and thoughts alone that goes with the word "chemotherapy." Thoughts and thoughts alone. That's cognition and cognition alone.

Well it's an ultimate— I mean, it's a seri— it's a number of antimetabolites whose property is to delay mitosis, abnormal mitosis, as much as possible, and therefore preventing the formation of tumor, and— malignant or otherwise. It essentially— it has also other side effects associated to it, but it's main function is to be an antimetabolite. There is a side effect associated to it— varying in intensity and— and vary upon— vary as a result of the kinds of chemicals that are going given to me.

Are you nauseated right now?

Not really when I was talking.

Mm-hm. How about right now?

'S better. I just thought back to—

What—?

I mean, thinking about it doesn't bother me. I mean, I really can think about it.

Note that when he started thinking about chemotherapy, the nausea subsided. I will return to this phenomenon later to show how it can be used clinically. Let us continue with this patient:

You are going to get, in the affective channel, and only the affective channel. Not the channel of pure body sensation, and not the channel of cognition; do you understand. Solely affective channel. You are going to get the affect that goes with the word "chemotherapy." Now.

(Long pause) It's anxious.

Anxious.

Oh yes. Scared. Really scared. I mean just scared. (Long pause.) Just scared.

Why are you scared. What are you scared of?

Fee—

Hm?

Well, I have to go into thoughts then. And— and—

No— What other affect of scared are you? Where are you scared? How are you scared?

I am scared of a recurrence.

That's what I meant.

As this dialogue demonstrates, not only does a word evoke thoughts and somatic sensations, it also brings forth an emotional response. And, as the next example indicates, words have at least one more dimension of meaning—the transcendent.

Now we are putting in the channel of religion. Religious channel. And only the religious channel. Not affective, not cognitive, not sensation. The religious channel that goes with the word "surgery."
For Christ sakes, let's hope it's working out. Will work out.
Is there such a thing as a religious channel?
Oh yes.
Is there?
Oh yes.
And what is it like when the word goes to the religious channel?
Oh, to me it's really— It's the most important channel. It's the least— expressible one. Because there's so much confusion about it. But it's also, to me, the most real one. I mean, one of the most real ones. Because I think that— I just think that it is! And— and it's not expressible with words or with thinking or with sensation or with any of those channels. It's something that transcends you and me.
Do you— It produced that in you when I said that?
Yes.

For the same patient, and in the same interaction, another word:

And in that religious channel again, and only the religious channel, you are going to get the religious playback that goes with the word "cancer."
Oh— Eh— You see (long pause). Huh! Gee. (long pause) Hm!— Well, Job— Job, is a very good analogy. Because during all the time that he was losing his field, his cattle, health, friends, everything, he kept, nevertheless, believing in God. So do I. Notwithstanding the fact that cancer has its— I mean, I just don't know why. I don't want to know why, and I don't think it's useful to know why. And yet— I mean, in the final analysis, it's all in His hands, you know, so—

On that occasion, the first in which it had occurred to me to look for that particular "channel" of meaning, I used the word "religious." This dimension might also be termed the transcendant or spiritual meaning of a word. Respondents often have the same difficulty expressing what they are experiencing as did this man. Whatever it is seems, somehow, ineffable. All of us have had experiences where we felt part of something larger than ourselves—religion, patriotism, even team spirit may evoke the awareness of a greater dimension.

Perhaps there are other dimensions of meaning as well, still to be uncovered.

I have shown that words have not only cognitive and affective meanings but are also capable of producing somatic sensations and of evoking a spiritual awareness that the subject may find difficult to put into language. Although here the four dimensions of word meaning have been presented separately, in everyday life they are all mixed together. When you speak to someone, you are speaking to the person's body. You are also simultaneously speaking to the person's emotions and thinking function as well the listener's spiritual side. Before going on, let me illustrate these points with additional examples. This next subject is a fourth-year medical student, and this conversation was recorded just before graduation. She was, as is so often the case, anxious about her approaching internship. (Let me repeat that all of these examples are of people in a hypnotic trance.)

I want to know what the word means in the channel of cognition, thinking. In no other channel. The word—is "doctor."

A doctor is a person who takes care of you when you're sick.

OK. You can clear the channel now. You will now—hear the word only in the channel of affect. Doctor.

Well, I feel towards doctors like you would feel towards an authority figure with power, an...

What does that feel like? What's the emotion feel—like?

Someone that you admire and trust.

All right, we'll clear that channel. You're going to have this word only in the channel of body sensation—alone. Doctor.

Pain!

Where?

Everywhere.

You felt pain? Where did you feel pain?

In my arms, in my legs.

OK. You're going to have this meaning only in the channel of transcendence, spirituality, religion—whatever you want to call it. Only in that channel. Doctor!

Omnipotent beings. The doctor's like the Buddha.

But what does it feel like inside you.?

The doctor's the almighty, the all-knowing.

Shall we try another word in the channel of . . . transcendence? Intern!

The first word that comes to mind is, "Yeuch!" On—the spiritual side the intern is a fool who doesn't know what the heck he's doing and is a jerk. He thinks he knows something.

In the channel of affect for "intern," she replied, "fear." For cognition she supplied the word "scutdog." For somatic sensation she answered "pain." This young woman has a very different conception for the word "doctor" than she has for the word "intern." Incidentally the reason pain came up in both contexts was that she believed both physicians and interns cause their patients pain. With physicians, the pain necessarily occurs as the patient is made better. She believed that interns, however, were the source of much unnecessary pain. One is not surprised that she approached her internship with apprehension.

Let me continue in a somewhat lighter vein. The next subject is an accomplished young philosopher who is about to start teaching a course on the philosopher Hegel for the first time.

. . . I can tell you you're going to hear the word and you're going to have a meaning for it in a channel—we'll call "body sensation." HEGEL. What's that . . . feel like?

Nervous! (Nervous laugh.) Sick! Aaaaj!

That's all right. Now relax again. In just a few moments you're going to hear a word, and its going to have meaning in the channel of cognition, thinking,—and only thinking. HEGEL.

A nineteenth-century German philosopher who wrote *The Phenomenology of Mind* . . . Its a litany, shall I go on?

You're going to hear the word again, and its going to have an effect for you only in the channel of affect and only affect. Emotion. HEGEL.

FEAR!

In the "channel" of transcendence for the name, Hegel, she found "everything clear and extremely nice."

Once again a word—in this case the name of a philosopher whose work she was about to teach, and whom she respected highly—had meanings in all four dimensions. The content of her conception for the word "Hegel" was extremely rich and many faceted and was not confined to merely intellectual content, or even cognitive plus emotional meanings. There were, in addition, both somatic sensations and transcendent experience associated with the word. The various aspects of meaning may not be congruent. In her case, as in so many other instances, the meanings at different levels were at odds with one another. The emotion of fear and the somatic sensation of anxiety are similarly negative, while the transcendant feelings were positive. When we know that she is about to teach her first graduate course on Hegel's work, it is not surprising that she has fear associated with the word, although, perhaps, not with Hegel's thinking.

It is this dynamic quality of meaning that is so difficult to grasp in discussions of the function of language. Words in dictionaries are static. And even when we are aware that meanings change, words continue to have an almost structural quality. The problem of understanding the function of language is akin to other structure-function issues in medicine. Look at a skeleton and an anatomy book picture of a group of muscles. Then attempt to picture the two—bones and muscles—in action in the living organism. It is a difficult task. The transition from static object, like muscles in a picture or words in a dictionary, to the dynamic process that is human physiology or human verbal communication is extremely difficult to accomplish.

Words also have individual meanings of which the person is unaware and, in addition, is unable to call to awareness in the ordinary course of events. These, often called "unconscious," meanings have been attached to the words during the course of life experience. Often the experiences associated with unconscious word meanings occurred in early childhood, but that need not be the case. I have avoided extensive reference to word meanings that are either unconscious or have symbolic meaning totally unique to the individual speaker. Listeners cannot usually know the speaker's deep or unconscious meanings, they can only know what the person says. Beyond this, listeners are forced to presumption or speculation. In the present era more is often made of listening with the "third" ear than with the other two. I have frequently had students and physicians tell me that, although the patient did not actually say so, a certain deep symbolic association was implied. How could they know for certain? Were they prepared to act on such evidence? I believe, however, that it has been demonstrated that such unconscious mechanisms not only exist but often determine human behavior—in sickness and in health.

How can I reconcile my failure to address unconscious meanings more directly with my belief in their importance? In this book I have attempted to provide tools that will allow a trained listener to hear what the patient is saying and what the patient means at every level of meaning. These tools, however, require you to document your conclusions from the direct evidence of the speaker's utterance. Even when deeper meanings are not immediately evident, they make their presence known in the paralanguage, word choice, logical structure, and syntax used by the speaker. These observable clues provide the listener with both the opportunity and the techniques to pursue additional meanings that may not be immediately apparent. I am aware, however, that with experience, one begins to know what people mean after very little evidence. But in these instances (which often sound like mind reading to less practiced observers), the experienced listener can, by asking a few questions, often make the evidence to support the interpretation explicit. I remember seeing an adolescent who was worried that there must be something wrong with his penis. His complaint was that he often had a split urinary stream. I found nothing, but I happened to mention the incident to an experienced psychiatrist who said, "Its probably masturbation guilt." The psychiatrist was correct, as I was able to ascertain when I next saw the young man. This incident has always seemed to me to represent the kind of arcane, but very useful, knowledge of human behavior that experienced physicians acquire. A few questions could bring the information to light, and the logical connection was clear: the urinary stream is split by dried seminal fluid remaining in the distal urethra or at the meatus.

The next example shows how meanings become attached to an object, event, or relationship and how the word for the thing can serve as the link that brings the meanings and associations to the surface. This forty-three-year-old woman, an artist, had recurrent herpes vulvovaginitis, the episodes of which she and her psychiatrist were convinced were evoked by specific emotional events. In this example, she has been hypnotized and is responding to the word "herpes."

_____

Now, it is the case that a word can come right in your ear and go in different channels. There is the channel of thought—of thinking, of moving facts around. And there's a channel for feeling, and emotions and affect. And there's a channel for body sensations that words can go to. And there's maybe even another channel that doesn't even have a name. And we're going to take a word, just for the fun of it, and see where the word goes. And then we'll be able to find out the definition of things. The word is "herpes." In the channel of body sensation and body sensation alone, let "herpes" go. Now!! What is that sensation?

It's a pulsation.

And where is that pulsation?

In the pelvic area.

Is that a pleasant or an unpleasant thing?

It's just there.

And is that the usual feeling that you have in your body and your body alone when you have herpes?

Unconsciously.

And consciously you have a different one?

Mm-hm.

But we'll stay with where the word goes, right? Pulsation. In your pelvis. And we'll let that pulsation get stronger and stronger. And feel it and sense it in the body and the body alone. Describe it better.

It's—it goes uh, it just beats. Just like that. Like a drum.

We'll take that sensation now, and hang it over there, on the wall, to use again when we need to know more about it . . . . Then we'll let the word, "herpes" go right back into the channel of thought and only thought.

Jeffry.

Jeffry?? More, please. Jeffry is a thought. Jeffry is a fact.

Jeffry's a name.

Thought. Don't stop. Thought.

It's hard.

If it's hard, we'll put it aside. Shall we do that? All right. Thought and thought alone.

Birth— Guess that's genital enough. It feels . . . (Later) Hate. I hate it.

What's that feel like, Sara?

It's the same hate I feel about herpes. I hate— what does it feel like? It feels angry, and it feels . . . blue.

Why those words, those images, those feelings? Blue, huh?

Blue's a color. Blue's color is icy and it's the antithesis of something warm and sunny. It's steely. I guess it's the way I felt on a February night when it was very cold in the cabin when I gave birth to Jeffry. Felt like that. I didn't feel angry, I didn't feel hate. I felt very cold, very blue.

In the cabin? Jeffry was born without a doctor?

Mm-hm.

We'll come back. We have one more channel. Unnamed. An unnamed channel. The only place left to go for that word that is neither thought, nor feeling, nor body sensation; Herpes!

It's just a word that screams at me.

From where?

I want to say "from out there," wherever "out there" is.

Well, from heaven or earth or hell or where?

I guess it could do with punishment. I guess, I— um, got the herpes after the accident. Which I don't consider an accident. I got the herpes after the trauma of the operation on the knee, which I really I trusted Jeffry, on that Skidoo, to know what he was doing because he said he knew what he was doing. And I followed his instructions. We all did. And from later, from knowledge, it was a totally made up set of instructions. It had nothing to do with the real . . . reality of Skidooing. I trusted him and he didn't know what he was talking about, and I trusted him knowing that he's not trustworthy in these areas. So I was very angry at him for being the way he was. And I was very angry at myself for putting everybody in jeopardy like that. My fantasy would be that my child would be perfect, and of course he would be totally reliable, and that anybody who says such a thing with such assurance you know he's done a hundred times before. But I knew underneath it all that he wasn't perfect, that he wasn't trustworthy, and I trusted him. And that was very poor judgment on my part. When I was very angry—I was angry at me; I was angry at him. And I'm angry for his imperfection. I'm angry that he's causing the problems that he's causing, the disturbances in my life at this point. I guess I go back to certain amounts of— These feelings about the birth were, ones of great up-ness, actually. I felt— I thought it had something to do with my doing it myself and that was going to make it all better. You know, he was going to be more perfect because I did it all by myself, and nobody had anything to do with the birthing but me. And I guess maybe I'm punishing myself for being punished, because certainly at this particular point in his life he is turning out to be a big pain in the ass.

What the herpes has to do— I felt cold that night, when I had him. I guess it has to do with the fact that I was doing something better than everybody else and therefore it was going to produce something that was better than everybody. It's back to my Perfect Image. Maybe I just haven't given up that. I also have— I've been having a lot of trouble separating from him. I'm very angry at him.

(Later)

And we will take a throbbing back off the wall and put it on you. We hung it there before, so that now you are throbbing, like you did before. And you'll let that throbbing grow and grow and grow, and then you'll know—what that is. That throbbing?

It's a birthing.

It's a birthing?!!

Because I didn't hurt when I birthed, either. Not really. I never had any real pain with it. It was a sensation, and it was strong, but it wasn't painful. Herpes is painful. This throbbing is different. It's like birthing. At least it was that way with Jeffry. It wasn't that way with Kimball . . .

The string of associations that have been set off by the word "herpes" are probably not accessible to her in states of ordinary consciousness. It would be highly unusual, however, if this patient did not offer clues to the doctor caring for her vulvovaginitis that the herpetic recurrences had begun to acquire secondary meanings. Whether her physician chose to follow up the clues is another matter. Too often patients are referred for psychotherapy because of persistent symptoms or illnesses, simply because the primary physician is at a loss as to what to do next. While understandable, such referrals are, I believe, more helpful when they are based on information elicited during conversations between the patient and primary physician than they are when they merely represent actions equivalent to throwing one's hands up in the air. In such conversations it is not necessary that the physician find out in detail what repressed emotional material has become attached to the illness. Uncovering the association would be difficult since the information has been repressed in order to protect the patient against the anxiety or other emotion that would follow self-discovery. It is much easier simply to demonstrate to the patient how much unhappiness, fear, anxiety or other painful emotion has become attached to the illness, and how the patient might be helped by psychotherapy, even if the illness itself cannot be cured. (Incidentally, referrals for psychotherapy are also more effective when the primary physician assures the patient that he or she is not being abandoned or "sent away"; that the doctor will always be there when needed.)

What a long and complicated road we have followed starting from the denotative, dictionary, meaning of a word. The meaning of words, it turns out, are as rich and complex as the world they represent for persons. Let me see if I can retrace our route. The place to start is by making it clear that words, signs, and symbols have both public and private functions. Speakers communicate not only with others but with themselves. And the "others" are not all alike. Speech and language must serve to communicate with total strangers as well as with lifelong intimates. A speech community is not a unitary body. There is the speech community of international pilots who use English to communicate with each other and with airport towers—even though an individual pilot may not be a native English speaker. There are the speech communities called "the United States," "New York," "doctors," "New York doctors," "renal dialysands," and endless others, that cross, contain, interact; each has claim on a portion of the internal content a speaker has for a particular word. It is clear that the highly individual portions of the inner content associated with words or expressions are *not necessary* for everyday public conversation. Indeed, if everyone who spoke to the woman with recurring pleural effusion knew that her pleural effusion evoked thoughts of spermatozoa, and that she hated sex, they would be mightily discomfited. Such knowledge, however, is very useful to some of those who treat her (as well as to those with whom sex was part of her interaction).

If language is as necessary to thought as is commonly believed, then a person's communication with self can, and probably does, utilize every individual nuance of meaning. And, as we have seen, such communication with self implies effects on emotions, on bodily sensations or the body itself, on spiritual aspects of being, as well as the more commonly assumed cognitive functions. Further, as every reader can immediately verify, thinking (in words) goes on while people listen to a speaker. Indeed, everyone is familiar with the phenomenon of listening to someone and then going off on another train of thought even though the speaker continues talking; indeed, breaking that habit is one of the difficult parts of becoming a trained listener. When you are the speaker, you recognize that the listener is not paying as much attention by the fact the listener's eyes shift away from yours into some other space. Unless they are bored—not usually the case when patients listen to their doctors talk about them—listeners are thinking about what they are hearing. From what has gone before in this chapter, *it should be clear that the patient's train of thought about what the doctor is saying may have meanings—from the cognitive to the transcendental—widely at odds with what the doctor means.* The question for the doctor is whether he or she wants the patient to hear the doctor's meaning or the patient's own meanings, especially since the doctor probably has a better idea of his or her own meanings than of what the same words mean to the patient.

This next example is an oncologist talking to a patient about chemotherapy. Read it with the example of the man who told us about the meanings of chemotherapy in the various channels in mind. It is a classic example of vague reference. This is unfortunately the way most physicians speak to patients about serious matters.

I gotta give you some more medicine my friend.

Yeah, I know.

So just, ah, hang on, and we'll start the chemotherapy on you today, you'll get it through today, so you'll get it Friday, Saturday, Sunday, Monday, Tuesday, then we'll be just about done and by the time I come back here, I hope you'll have finished the third course and then we'll be through with you. Now we may— if the medicine doesn't work this time around, what I'm going to have to do is switch off to a different medicine to try to get this thing licked. But we've got to get— we've got to get all these cells cleaned out because if we don't get these cells cleaned out, we're just going to be behind the eight ball and we'll be beating our head against a stone wall. So it's very important that we try to get these cells cleaned out, and I'm going to give you a third dose of medicine. Then after that we'll start talking about something else. I hope this third dose is going to do the trick. OK?

Yeah.

All right, so just hang on there and I hope everything works out for you all right. Your temperature's down so you must be feeling a little bit better.

Yeah.

Many physicians, on hearing this example, are chagrined because this is exactly the way they talk. We are all afraid of telling patients things that are painful, or difficult, or frightening, so we choose words that are deliberately vague. When you speak vaguely, however, you do not avoid bad meanings; instead you give the patient the opportunity to use his or her own interpretation. And, though not invariably so, in serious disease the patient's meanings are almost always worse, full of terrible fear, awful thoughts, nausea, anxious muscle tightness, and even, sometimes, impending doom. Even worse, the same reaction may be evoked in minor illness when explanations are vague, because it is a habit of our speech community that speakers most often avoid direct reference when they are discussing matters that are best avoided: serious outcomes such as blindness (opthalmologists take notice), permanent crippling (orthopedists and rheumatologist pay attention), disfigurement (attention dermatologists), or death (we must all take notice here).

This next example comes from MacIntosh's book about doctor-patient communication on a cancer ward in Great Britain, which was published in 1979:

You've got a bit of thickening there. We'll take a bit of it out and have a look at it under the microscope and, if there are any suspicious cells there, we'll have to do a more radical procedure. Even if there's a small chance that there might be, we'll have to remove your breast just to be sure.

When we take you to theatre, we'll take a bit of this out and have a look at it under the microscope and, if any of the cells look as if they might become nasty, we will remove the breast. We always try to err on the side of safety.

How things have changed! This is the way New York physicians spoke to their patients about carcinoma of the breast in the 1950s. Nowadays no one could get away with a conversation like that. Every American woman knows that one does not have a mastectomy unless one has carcinoma. Further many women have formed opinions about which operation they think is best for them! Why did those British physicians speak in that manner? There is one very practical reason. When one is vague enough, one has no fear of being contradicted by what the next doctor says. Thus such conversations have the advantage of uniformity of message. But that is not the overriding reason, as the monograph from which the conversation comes makes clear. The physicians believed that if the patient knew she had cancer, she would feel doomed and lose hope. Further, having hope is considered so important that the uncertainty created by their message is believed less important. (Despite the importance attached to the word "hope," the book gave no evidence of attempts to understand the concept of hope in the same manner as one might try and understand say the best incision for a mastectomy.) What the book *does* make clear is that most of the patients knew that they had cancer. Thus, while the cloud created by the physicians' statements did not keep that knowledge from the patients, it did create foreboding and uncertainty. In his book *The Trial*, Franz Kafka created an atmosphere of horror by surrounding his protagonist with uncertainties. "Who is accusing me? Of what am I accused? Who are these people? Where am I?" If you wish to create dread, helplessness, and hopelessness, it is best done by surrounding a patient with uncertainties. "What is the matter with me? What is going to happen to me? Why won't my doctor tell me anything?" This is the atmosphere that may be created by vague reference.

What I have demonstrated in this chapter suggests that not only does open and direct communication by a physician avoid the dangers of vague reference, but that it has a positive effect of its own. What happened to the patient describing the cognitive meaning of chemotherapy? His nausea disappeared. If you talk directly to people about what is happening in their body using detailed facts that are understandable, they start to feel better. Carefully explaining why the pulmonary embolus caused the pleural effusion, and how that produced the pain, and what the anticoagulants do, and so on, the more detailed the better (so long as it is understandable), begins to make the patient feel better—and feeling better is part of being better. Actually, the fact that shifting to a cognitive mode dulls body sensation is common knowledge in sexual situations. Talking to someone who is in pain about the pain itself, how it is produced, what body mechanisms are involved, and what will happen to it, produces pain relief once the patient starts paying attention.

It is because people often magically equate the word for something with the thing itself that diagnostic statements can be therapeutic. How words do their therapeutic work is another matter entirely. In the introduction to my book *The Healer's Art*, there is a description of my "talking" an older woman out of pulmonary edema. In the situation in which the patient and I found ourselves, a psychiatric ward in the old Bellevue Hospital, there were no drugs or oxygen. All I could do was talk. I told her about pulmonary edema in all the detail I could, all the while assuring her that the fluid level would go down—which, to my surprise, is exactly what happened. I did not understand the phenomenon then, and I am not sure I do now, but this chapter suggests some possible mechanisms. You will rapidly be able to demonstrate these mechanisms for yourself.

This next illustration is a surgeon explaining bypass surgery to a patient in the cardiac intensive care unit. As you will note, the surgeon is not only complete but makes use of visual aids.

Well, it's pretty much the way Dr. Cassell and Dr. Rinditi thought it was going to be. You have— well, you know you have had a heart attack in the past. And it looks as if things are getting set up for you to have another one. And our job right now is to try and prevent this from happening. The fact that you've began having pain—

You mean the blood vessels in the heart, the coronary arteries—in the heart—constricts?

Yeah. One of the blood vessels is quite— narrow. And it's a very important blood vessel. This is why the study was done this morning, to see WHICH blood vessel or predictably SOMETHING was—

Mm-hm.

—either happening or about to happen.

So what are my options.

I think what all of us are going to recommend is that you have an operation. And that you have it tomorrow morning.

And what's that? For cleaning out the arteries?

No. Oh no. Put a bypass around the artery that's blocked. I drew a little picture here of your artery. That's sort of diagrammatically what the problem is. These are the major arteries that supply blood to the heart. This blood vessel here, is totally blocked. And this is one of what we call the three major ones. This one, this, one, and that one, are the three major ones. This one is totally blocked and probably has been totally blocked for a long time. That probably happened when you had your heart attack in the past.

Mm-hm.

This one is a large blood vessel in you, and is a very significant blood vessel, and it has a little bit of narrowing in it but nothing of any real significance. The very significant finding in your study this morning was that in this blood vessel here which comes right off and supplies the entire side of the left side of your heart— this is about ninety-five percent plus, narrowed. And I think this is what is responsible for your having this accelerated—

Right.

—problem at the present time. What we propose to do about this is— there's very little we can do about this one that's totally blocked.

Yeah.

What's done is done. There's very little we can do to bring that back. But we can put a conduit, a piece of vein that we'll take from your leg, around this blocked area here and to an artery beyond that so we can bypass this. It's like a detour. Bypass where the bridges are.

All right, I got it.

Visual aids make the task easier, but the possibility is created in the first place by the function of words, signs, and symbols.

If this chapter has been successful, it should have enlarged your understanding, not only of how words work, but of the therapeutic possibilities of the spoken language.

References

MacIntosh, Jim. *Communication and Awareness in a Cancer Ward.* New York: Prodist, 1977.

Cassell, Eric J. *The Healer's Art.* New York: Lippincott, 1976. Penguin, 1980.

6

An Everyday Language of Description

One time I took care of a very obstructive, demanding, querulous, old, and very wealthy man following his prostatic surgery. He was weak to the point of being bedridden prior to his operation, and his weakness worsened postoperatively. For many years he had been accustomed to having others do everything for him, and it was maddeningly difficult to coax him to turn, cough, or even breathe for himself. I believe he owed his survival not to the servants that crowded his room, but to the stubborn, yet gentle efforts of the subintern who was insistent that he live. When she rotated off service, she wrote a note in his chart that exactly depicted his personal characteristics and the qualities required to get him to perform. When I complimented her on the description, the equal of which I had not seen in a hospital chart, and told her how important it was to be able describe patients in that fashion, she said, "I didn't write it as a doctor. He was so difficult that I thought if the next person taking over knew what he was like, it would be much easier. I don't think I could write a medical description like that. I would freeze up!"

Sad as it is, she is correct; doctors do not seem to be able to portray what their patients are like. If you open the charts of people I have taken care of for over twenty years, nowhere in that considerable volume of material will you find a description of the patients. Some momentous things have happened to them, but the only clues you will have concerning how the patients have been changed by their diseases and illnesses are those given by the pathology and X-ray reports, laboratory sheets, and other weights and measures. But it is my intimate knowledge of them—what kind of people they are, how they have behaved in sickness, and the nature of their relationships with others—in addition to my technical knowledge, that allows me to be effective when they require care. In common with other physicians, I carry that information in my head. If a patient changes physicians or moves away, the next doctor must start fresh to learn about the person, although information about the body is contained in the copy of the chart that I transmit. What a waste.

There is of course one very practical reason for this deficiency of my patient records, and the same defect in virtually every hospital and office record I have ever seen. Nobody ever taught us! Although some understanding of what a patient is like is essential to the care of almost every patient by every doctor, such information has not previously been considered part of *medical* knowledge. I am not being entirely fair. One does see renderings of patients' emotional states. From reading them, one would get the impression that everybody is either anxious or depressed. Lately, parsimony has been introduced into that thin lexicon and now one sees that patients have only a "negative" or "positive" affect. Occasionally a chart has an entry by a social worker or a psychiatrist which is manifestly about the person of the patient. But, with exceptions, between abbreviations and technical jargon, it is difficult to recognize who they are writing about. Nobody ever seems to be sad, unhappy, sulky, gloomy, moody, mean, or even, happy, high-strung, jumpy, enthusiastic, quick-tempered, and so on. In attempting to exclude value judgments from descriptive statements, we have gone so far as to make our descriptions valueless! We must be able to do better.

It is truly said that if you cannot describe something, you do not know about it. Throughout this book, it is stressed that the attentive listener hears not only what the speaker's narrative tells but also what the speaker is like, as suggested by language choice. It follows that unless you begin to learn a language of description, you may not be about to utililize fully the information available from the patient. It is certainly the case that you will not be able to share your knowledge with others in the absence of a common language of description.

When medical students are taught physical diagnosis, they are also taught a descriptive language that will serve to record their findings and communicate them to other doctors. An acutely arthritic joint is "red, hot, swollen, and tender." If I add "exquisitely tender," you may begin to suspect a septic joint, or gout. But if I write those findings—including "exquisite"—about the big toe, then you will almost certainly think first of gout. That interpretation (often wrong) is implied by the word picture. There lies a problem with any language of description: it should provide a representation, not an interpretation or conclusion. But "fluffy white spots," or "flame shaped red spots," about an eyeground are descriptive without leading the reader. In a similar fashion "lemon yellow" or "orangy yellow" conjunctivae clearly picture different degrees of jaundice. I can go on to talk about wounds that are "red, swollen, and puckered around the sutures," or pus that has a "fecal odor," or even "tympanitic abdomen" to make the point that in comparison with physicians' usual ability to portray persons, our language of description for physical phenomena is rich and communicative, allowing the reader or listener to visualize what the observer is characterizing without necessarily subscribing to the observer's conclusions.

The genius of the disease theory is that it finally provided a basis for doctors to talk about sick persons using a commonly agreed on language. Angina pectoris, coronary heart disease, rheumatic mitral valvular disease, oat cell carcinoma of the lung, and immune complex syndromes have common meanings wherever western medicine is practiced. The advantages that common terminology can provide for research and therapeutics cannot be overemphasized. It has taken one hundred and fifty years to achieve such unanimity of terms. (However, it requires frequent national and international conferences to maintain common language usage because of the natural drift in language practice.) Such linguistic precision became possible when doctors could not only agree on the words but also on the defining characteristics of the diseases indicated by their names. Psychiatric nomenclature has suffered from the lack of preciseness and agreed on definitions, and that is one (but only one) of the reasons for the deep schisms between different schools of thought in psychiatry and between psychiatrists and nonpsychiatrists. Finding a language of description for patients will certainly present difficulties if we require total agreement on the definitions and nomenclatures portraying the different types of people. It simply cannot be done.

An example from another discipline in medicine may offer guidance. British and American epidemiologists did not agree on the definition of chronic bronchitis. The usual way in which such problems are solved, by first reaching agreement on the anatomic pathology, did not help. Even microscopic anatomy failed to provide grounds for unanimity. Then it turned out that the distinction between emphysema and chronic bronchitis collapsed. There was one finding, however, that was the same for British patients, whose lung troubles satisfied the criteria of British physicians, and American patients, who had chronic obstructive lung disease to the satisfaction of American doctors: they both answered questions about cough and phlegm the same way. Since the definitive questions were in everyday language, so now is the current definition of chronic obstructive lung disease. Patients who cough and produce phlegm on most days for as much as three months a year, and have done so for at least two years, have, by definition, chronic obstructive pulmonary disease! When that definition was advanced, it was unique in medicine, partly because of its use of everyday language. (It has subsequently been possible to find physiologic abnormalities common to those who have chronic cough and phlegm.)

I think the solution to the problem of describing persons for medical practice is to use everyday language. Unfortunately that does not end the problem. For example, to say that a patient is "nasty, churlish, and mean," or, conversely, "a heaven-sent delight," certainly uses everyday language, but it does not solve the problem of definitions. What is the meaning of "churlish"? I do not believe we could all agree on the characteristics of "a heaven-sent delight." Such characterizations are often a matter of taste or result from life experiences. Because of the subjectivity of such words—because they are really words of opinion—they will not serve the purpose of descriptions of person for medical practice.

We need a model to point the way, and novelists would seem to be our best guides. Descriptive language is the writer's stock and trade, and Charles Dickens was among the best at its use. On the first page of *Dombey and Son,* Mr Dombey and his newborn son are described:

Dombey was about eight-and-forty years of age. Son was about forty-eight minutes. Dombey was rather bald, rather red, and though a handsome well-made man, too stern and pompous in appearance to be prepossessing. Son was very bald, and very red, and . . . somewhat crushed and spotty in his general effect . . . On the brow of Dombey, Time and his brother Care had set some marks . . . while the countenance of Son was crossed and recrossed with a thousand little creases . . . Dombey . . . jingled and jingled the heavy gold watch-chain that extended from below his trim blue coat . . .

In those few phrases we are given the outward appearance of Dombey, a London merchant. In addition we are told he is pompous. But Dicken does not simply say Dombey is pompous, he allows readers to come to the same conclusion by providing a word portrait that fits a pompous man. Suppose, for instance, that Dombey had been "tall, fine-featured, with intense eyes that, like their owner, moved quickly . . ." After such a depiction the author could not have said that Dombey was pompous, our own experience would not support his conclusion. Thus an effective description, even when it contains an interpretation, provides the evidence to back it up. Here is a portrayal of Miss Tox:

The lady thus presented was a long lean figure, wearing such a faded air that she seemed not to have been made in what linen-drapers call "fast colours" originally, and to have, little by little, washed out. But for this she might have been described as the very pink of general propitiation and politeness. From a long habit of listening admirably to everything that was said in her presence, and looking at speakers as if she were mentally engaged in taking off impressions of their images upon her soul, never to part with the same but with life, her head had quite settled on one side. Her hands had contracted a spasmodic habit of raising themselves of their own accord as an involuntary admiration. Her eyes were liable to a similar affection. She had the softest voice that ever was heard; and her nose, stupendously acquiline, had a little knob in the very centre or key-stone of the bridge, whence it tended downwards towards her face, as an invincible determination never to turn up at anything.

Miss Tox's dress, though perfectly genteel and good, had a certain character of angularity and scantiness. She was accustomed to wear odd weedy little flowers in her bonnets and caps. Strange grasses were sometimes perceived in her hair; and it was observed by the curious, of all her collars, frills, tuckers, wristbands, and other gossamer articles—indeed of everything she wore which had two ends to it intended to unite—the two ends were never on good terms, and wouldn't quite meet without a struggle. She had furry articles for winter wear, as tippets, boas, and muffs, which stood up on end in a rampant manner, and were not at all sleek. She was much given to the carrying about of small bags with snaps to them, that went off like little pistols when they were shut up; and when full-dressed, she wore round her neck the barrenest of lockets, representing a fishy old eye, with no approach to speculation in it. These and other appearances of a similar nature had served to propagate the opinion that Miss Tox was a lady of what is called a limited independence, which she turned to the best account. Possibly her mincing gait encouraged the belief, and suggested that her clipping a step of ordinary compass into two or three originated in her habit of making the most of everything.

I do not know Miss Tox, and neither do you, but I think that we can agree that she will not be the patient who openly argues with her doctor. It is possible, however, that in order to save money, she might not have a prescription filled unless her doctor had made its necessity absolutely clear (and even, perhaps, implied that not to get the medication and take it as directed would be an expression of dis-respect). She seems a bit odd, however, and so we must be prepared for the unexpected and be cautious in prejudging. But with the awareness created by what we *do* know, we will watch closely, ask questions especially carefully and listen attentively when she speaks. Within a few visits we will be able to take care of her very much better, and she will, with reason, feel understood.

Notice that much of what we have come to know of Miss Tox in those paragraphs comes from a description of her behavior—Miss Tox is pictured *in action*. If we were merely told that she is long and lean, or that her nose is "stupendously acquiline," such language, although unquestionably descriptive, would not reveal what kind of a person *she* is. Physical characteristics alone would provide an image not unlike early daguerreotypes—frozen and unnatural. The addition of behaviors rounds out the characterization. But the conduct of Miss Tox that Dickens writes about is merely bearing, demeanor, mannerisms, and habit of dress. From these small pieces of the total Miss Tox we form an impression that supports speculation about some behaviors as quite possible for her and others as improbable. In general, even to know as little as we are told about Miss Tox provides an enormous amount of information about a total person. The reason is that people, in their dress, demeanor, gait, speech, facial expression, activities, work, in all of the characteristics that make up their persons, are *more*, rather than less, consistent.

Caution is necessary in interpreting and acting on the last statement. Leaving aside prevalent preconceptions concerning the era about which Charles Dickens writes, can we guess what kind of sexual partner Miss Tox might be? Absolutely not. Some aspects of a person, such as sexual behavior, private fantasies, what is done in the intimacy of the home, or behavior during life-threatening illness, are not even open to educated speculation without very much more knowledge of the individual because it is in the nature of humankind that those behaviors may *not* be consistent with the manner in which the self is presented in everyday life. These aspects of the person *can* be known, if necessary, by asking about them.

Further, interpreting behaviors is open to the same error as interpreting speech: Is the doctor hearing what the *patient* means by an utterance, or what the *doctor* would mean if he or she said the same words? In interpreting behaviors, is the doctor making a judgment about the patient's conduct based on the patient's actions, or on what it would mean about the doctor if he or she behaved similarly? The error is avoided two ways. First, the observer should be aware of as many different details of speech, physical appearance, dress, and demeanor as possible. For doctors to decide what a patient is like based on what it would mean if *they* presented themselves in a similar fashion, unless they and the patient are absolutely identical, it would be necessary for them to disregard details inconsistent with their conclusions. As was discussed in chapter 2, part of the information that must be employed to know what a patient means by a particular word comes from the other words in the utterance; the values expressed in the modifying adjectives and adverbs, the degree of passivity or activity of the verbs, and the kinds of nouns and pronouns. The context of the conversation also plays a part in interpretation. So it is with the other aspects of the presentation of self—it is not one small detail alone on which judgments are based but on the totality of the evidence.

One must distinguish between the accuracy of the depiction of a patient and the correctness of the judgments based on it. The former depends on the acuteness of the observer, but judgment depends more on experience. In this regard what I am presenting is similar to the well-known difference between the accuracy of a test result and its diagnostic utility. While life experience is essential in order to become astute about people, acumen will develop much faster, I believe, in good observers than in those who have not trained their senses. As Montaigne noted long ago, Nature makes nothing that is not different than another. Thus it is that the mindful observer learns first how dissimilar everybody is. One may wonder how it is that knowing the almost infinite differences in the details of individuals could lead to astuteness in judgment. If everybody appeared the same, on what basis could one judge? Judgment, to be of value, must be based on evidence, and evidence presents itself as differences.

In learning to describe patients, physicians must rid themselves of a common habit of mind: the uneasiness that comes with making judgments about people; the sense that it is intrinsically "rude." Of course that is precisely what everyone (more or less privately) does—judge others. And most such opinions must be negative, else why would there be sanctions against them? In the course of my working day I do many things not generally considered polite. I put my fingers where people learn from childhood not to put their own hands, much less allow access to others. I ask questions about taboo subjects and tell patients things about themselves they do not want to hear. All this is accepted by society because it is in the service of others. I did not learn to be comfortable with these behaviors in a minute, though it started by eating lunch in the anatomy lab. Patients are greatly concerned that they look clean and that their feet not smell too badly. I no longer care about or look down on those with smelly feet or (with exceptions) unclean bodies, wounds, or diseases. Physicians learn to make judgments about people, interpret their actions, and predict their behavior without feeling that they have thus wronged the patients. On the contrary, it is done in their behalf.

One might object that doctors could be supreme patient describers if they had the time and space that Charles Dickens employed writing about Miss Tox. Here is another portrait: "A cheerful-looking merry boy, fresh with running home in the rain; fair-faced, bright-eyed, and curley haired." Dickens could be parsimonious when he wished. Again, it is the demeanor and behavior presented in those few words that makes the representation so effective. Let us see what the physician has the opportunity to observe in an initial interview: physical appearance, dress, makeup and ornamentation, demeanor, speech. This is an impressive array of features—certainly enough to characterize the manner in which a person presents him or herself in a physician's office. (Never forget that the presentation of self is, in part, context dependant, and a doctor's office or a hospital is a very special context.) With the exception of physical appearance, each facet is a *behavior*, not an architectural detail—even facial expression is an action. Few would disagree that accurate characterization of those aspects of human behavior would provide a good basis for representing an individual in words. What is required is a vocabularly of everyday language for description.

Because this book is primarily about the spoken language, in the remainder of the chapter I will provide a lexicon for portraying a person's speech—that is, their verbal behavior. Then I will offer a vocabulary of terms that can be used to record the impression of the person arising from a description of speech. There are several ways of employing this list. One way is to record several persons in conversation; even recordings of radio or television conversations will serve. Listen to the speaker, and then, category by category, choose the word that best fits what you hear. It may be that in the beginning most speakers will sound pretty much the same, but as you work along you will find that being forced to choose from among the descriptive words will itself sharpen your ears. If you had to decide what they sounded like without the vocabulary that I have provided, you would find it more difficult to portray the speaker's language. Although when we compiled this list, we attempted to be comprehensive, you may wish to add terms that better fit your representational powers. You are trying to develop your own language of description, something suitable to you and natural to your own style. I should caution you not to use abbreviations or, at least in the beginning, shorten the lists too much or you will end up with a "one-size-fits-all" descriptive language. That is the antithesis of the goal. As with all exercises of this kind, the more you practice the better you will be. After having worked with a tape recorder, take your list out in public. It is best to do that one category at a time. Start with the list for speech rate.

Listen to speakers and then tell yourself what term best describes their speech rate. Proceed to the remainder of the categories. Place the words on three by five cards and refer to them. Doing that with the voice quality list may represent a challenge, but medical students can do almost anything. *Expect the process of learning to take many months.* Unlike anatomy, which one must learn seven times and forget six, once you have acquired this skill, it will stay with you the remainder of your life. Indeed, within a year you will form your judgment almost automatically, although the evidence on which it is based will be available for recall. Remember, you are already making judgments about people, but they are generally uninformed by carefully collected facts! After having learned how to do this you may wish to make your own lists for facial expression, dress, makeup and ornamentation, and demeanor.

A. Paralanguage

1. Speech rate:

slow	rapid
leisurely	hurried
indolent	deliberate

2. Pause-speech rate ratio:

flowing	mechanical
rhythmic	halting
choppy	babbling
stuttering	staccato
long pauses, short pauses, no pauses, filled pauses, inappropriate pauses	

3. Tone or voice quality:

nasal	artificial
flat	whiney
dull	raspy
monotone	breathy
even	deep
bright or clear	gruff
cutting	gutteral
piercing	harsh
clipped	gravelly

mechanical
choked
smooth
soft
unctious
musical
singsong
emphatic

resonant
booming
feminine
masculine
strained
relaxed
babyish
husky

4. Pitch:
high   medium   low

5. Volume:
Loud
wide swings

quiet
even

6. Articulation:
precise
specific dialect differences

slurred

7. For all categories:
wide range of variations
rapid variation

B. Choice of words

accurate
precise
meticulous
pedantic
deliberate
technical
intellectual
elaborate
illiterate
poetic
metaphorical
flowery
exaggerated
bizarre

theatrical
formal
informal
thoughtful
careful
awkward
ordinary
colorful
simple
haphazard
chaotic
neologisms
repetitive
laborious

use of distancing mechanisms
(e.g., in choice of pronouns,
verb tense, or articles)

C. Sentence construction

elaborate   elliptical

simple   pedantic

awkward

syntactic distancing devices
(e.g., verb tense, temporal
ordering, use of negatives)

D. Logic

orderly

straightforward

consistent

complicated (containing multiple premises in a single utterance)

contradictory (containing premises that preclude each other)

ambivalent (containing multiple premises that contradict each other)

magical (containing premises whose truth would require magical powers)

childlike (imperfect connection of premises, as in "only a child would believe that")

confused or disjointed

unclear (making no attempt to establish common premises with a listener)

chaotic (premises presented in a seemingly random manner)

It is obvious that choosing from this list of descriptors allows for considerable individual variation. What, for example, is a "masculine" voice quality, and how is that different from "deep"? Why is "deep" on the list but not, say, "sonorous"? If you wish, put "sonorous" on the list and delete "masculine" and "feminine." You may use whatever words of depiction that you wish if they are drawn from everyday language and are employed in their usual meaning. Internal consistency is important. It would be difficult for me to imagine a speaker whose voice was "deep, sonorous, masculine, and babyish!"

One's first attempts at describing speakers are often so clumsy that it seems unlikely that fluency will develop. It will. In addition the problem of interpersonal differences diminishes with practice and with the awareness that word images are for *others*, not primarily for the observer. With that in mind, representational terms should be chosen to achieve maximum clarity. Practicing this technique with a group will aid in choosing terms that have meaning to others and avoiding usages whose depictive meaning is too idiosyncratic. Watch a television situation comedy with your friends, characterize the actors' speech, and then choose adjectives that best describe the character the actor is portraying. The advantage of sit-coms is that actors, by training, maintain constancy in their portrayal of characters, allowing you to practice on them week after week.

After the list of words that describe the person's speech has been compiled, it is time to characterize the individual in general terms. Adjectives are generally employed for this purpose. Unfortunately most doctors do not have a broad spectrum of adjectives ready at hand. Next you will find more than a hundred and fifty adjectives that have been drawn from a personality assessment tool known as the Adjective Check-List. (Copyright regulations have prevented me from presenting the entire three-hundred word list.) This psychological testing instrument has been extensively used and validated, and though we will not be applying these words for their original testing purpose, the device can be utilized to test students' progress in learning to listen. After hearing a recording of a patient presented during the first exercise of my course, I have requested students to describe the speaker in one sentence and by choosing adjectives from the check list. So varied were their responses that it is difficult to tell that they were all listening to the same person. In the last exercise of the course I repeated the demonstration. The results were gratifyingly different. It was apparent that they had learned to hear what kind of a person the speaker sounded like. Because the Adjective Check-List provides such a wide choice, allowance is made for individual differences in the choice of adjectives for essentially the same personality characterization. However, the scoring technique provided for the instrument will show if the person has been similarly considered, even though adjective choice varied between observers.

Instructors may wish to use the actual testing method as a means of measuring students' listening and observational abilities. The test sheets and scoring codes can be obtained from the company and can be scored automatically, if so desired.

Adjective Check-List*

absentminded	complaining	happy
active	complicated	hasty
adaptable	conceited	high-strung
adventurous	confident	honest
affected	confused	hostile
affectionate	conscientious	imaginative
aggressive	conservative	impatient
alert	considerate	impulsive
aloof	contented	independent
ambitious	conventional	indifferent
anxious	cool	informal
apathetic	cooperative	inhibited
appreciative	courageous	insightful
argumentative	cowardly	intelligent
arrogant	defensive	intolerant
artistic	demanding	irresponsible
assertive	dependent	irritable
attractive	despondent	logical
autocratic	determined	loud
awkward	dignified	mature
bitter	disorderly	mild
blustery	dissatisfied	modest
boastful	easygoing	moody
bossy	emotional	natural
calm	energetic	obliging
capable	enthusiastic	opinionated
careless	evasive	optimistic
cautious	excitable	outgoing
changeable	fair-minded	outspoken
charming	faultfinding	patient
cheerful	fearful	pessimistic
civilized	frank	pleasant
clear-thinking	frivolous	practical
clever	fussy	preoccupied
coarse	gloomy	prudish
cold	good-natured	quarrelsome
commonplace	handsome	realistic

reasonable	snobbish	tough
reckless	spontaneous	unaffected
relaxed	spunky	unassuming
resentful	stable	undependable
reserved	stern	unemotional
resourceful	stolid	unfriendly
restless	strong	ininhibited
retiring	suggestible	unkind
rude	sulky	unselfish
sarcastic	superstitious	unstable
self-controlled	suspicious	vindictive
sensitive	talkative	wary
sexy	tense	wise
shallow	thorough	withdrawn
shy	thoughtful	witty
simple	timid	worrying
slow	tolerant	

Let me illustrate how the description of speech fits with the list of adjectives. A fifty-two-year-old woman came to her physician to discuss placing her mother in a nursing home. Her speech was loud, high-pitched, and hurried with choppy pauses and a husky quality. Her word choice was exaggerated, but her sentences were straightforward. Scan the list of adjectives and see how many are *not* applicable to this woman with the information given. Of the first fifty-one adjectives, from "absentminded" to "cowardly," she might be aggressive, anxious, argumentative, assertive, blustery, or complaining. Indeed, she might be all of these, but the other forty-five adjectives do not apply. Here is another woman: her speech is moderately loud, deliberate, and rhythmic with an artificial quality. She precisely articulates her words, which, like her sentences, are elaborate and slightly theatrical. Again, only a few adjectives would fit a person so depicted. Incidentally, it would seem odd if this last woman had no makeup, wore an ill-fitting plain dress and brown flat shoes.

As you practice these technics remember that a description is good if someone else, reading it, can choose adjectives that correctly fit the person. The Adjective Checklist largely provides a language of *interpretation*, or conclusions. The lexicon for portraying speech, dress, physical appearance, and demeanor is a language of *observation*. When observations are detailed and accurate, and can be expressed clearly in everyday words, the major task is accomplished.

Appendix: Recording and Cataloging Doctor-Patient Communication

Nothing will enhance your communication skills so much as listening to tape recordings of yourself with patients. The utility of recordings, which are also effective aids to teaching, is enhanced if they are of high quality. When reproduction is poor, a listener is very much aware of hearing a recording. When, on the other hand, the sound is excellent, awareness is concentrated where it belongs, on the conversation. For the same reason stereophonic recordings are better than monophonic. These guidelines are written specifically for audio recording, but they apply equally to the sound quality of video recording.

Currently available equipment has put good cassette recordings within the practical reach of anyone who is interested, and the state of the art continues to improve. At the very least, then, one can place a small cassette recorder on the bed or desk between oneself and the patient and record the interaction.

Employing two "lapel" microphones greatly enhances the quality of the recording. In quiet surroundings the background noise diminishes and the voices achieve a lifelike clarity. In a noisy setting—one has only to start recording in hospital rooms to realize how much racket patients put up with—microphones may be required for the conversation to be intelligible. The quality of the microphones has much more effect on sound reproduction than the quality of tape recorders. Therefore, if money is limited, spend it on good microphones, not on fancy recorders. Sony ECM-50PS microphones are superb and cost at the time of this writing, $146.25. Not as good, but still excellent are Sony ECM-150 microphones which cost $48.75. Both of these microphones require batteries, but the ECM-50PS have longer-lasting batteries which are more convenient. Their wires are long enough to connect a microphone to the patient and one to yourself and still move easily about a hospital bed with the recorder on a bedside or overbed table, or in your pocket. The cords of the ECM-150 are shorter (extensions can be rigged), and you must pay attention to their batteries to ensure that they are "on" only when necessary or you will find, to your dismay, that you have failed to record because the batteries were dead or the microphone was turned off. Other manufacturers make similar products which, while not as good, will produce very satisfactory recordings. Because equipment has been improving so rapidly, when you read this there may be other, better, microphones that deserve a trial.

No matter how sophisticated or expensive the equipment, there are, alas no trouble-free or foolproof systems—vigilance is always required if one is to make decent recordings. The cassette must be properly inserted and the machine turned on! Checking the batteries regularly in both recorder and microphone is necessary and is facilitated by an inexpensive battery tester. Extra batteries should always be on hand. A checklist attached to the recorder can prevent many missed recordings. It is often practical and not difficult to make a small carrying case (I constructed mine from denim—it had a somewhat dashing look!) that holds the recorder, microphones, and a few spare parts, all readily accessible. Because machines are lighter these days, the entire setup is easily carried. (The one I originally employed was so heavy that I worried that one of the prices of the year-long research would be a shoulder separation!) Most of us when seeing patients in the office or hospital have other things on our minds besides taperecorders, consequently the setup should be as unobtrusive and convenient as possible. You will find that you do not make a recording even when you intended to if it is too much trouble. Once having decided to record interactions, it is a good idea to carry the recorder at all times. This way the patients and the staff all become accustomed to seeing the equipment as part of you, and it becomes relatively "invisible."

Explicit consent must be obtained before recording an interaction with a patient. It is not sufficient that the patient can see the recorder or the microphones and thus "understands" what is being done even though permission was not specifically requested. Written and signed consent forms are not necessary for informal recording. However, if the recordings are part of a research project, written consent may be required. In case of doubt ask your institutional review board. If the recordings, or any part of them are being played in public, used for teaching, or as part of lecture demonstrations, it is best to obtain written consent that specifically mentions these possibilities. For informal recording it is usually sufficient to say something like, "Mr.

Patient, may I have your consent to make a tape recording of our conversation. I am using these tapes to learn about doctor-patient communication. I will be listening to them myself, and your privacy will be respected." If you are employing them for other purposes, say so. The great majority of patients will give consent. Understandably the issue that usually concerns them is privacy. When the recordings on which this book is based were edited for teaching, the patients' and usually the doctors' names were removed. On the occasion when some tapes were employed on a radio program, we showed the patients transcripts of the conversation and requested written permission for the broadcast.

We employed a Revox reel-to-reel machine for recording an entire set of office hours or other similar prolonged period, because cassette recorders were inadequate. The Revox has ten-inch reels which allow, at three and three quarters inches per second, about three hours of recording before being turned over. The problem is microphone placement. In offices or treatment units where the doctor and patient remain in one small room, the common practice of suspending a microphone, which is usually not first rate, from the middle of the ceiling produces hollow sounding recordings that become indistinct when the voices are lowered or someone turns away. It is equally practical and far superior to employ "lapel" microphones on long cords. In larger units or in offices where the consulting room and examining rooms are separate, alternate procedures are necessary. We found that transmitting microphones produced the best recordings and were the most innocous for both doctor and patient. We made use of Sennheiser microphones, transmitters, and receivers which are expensive but excellent. The doctor carries the transmitter in a small pouch attached to the waist with the microphone clipped to the tie. The patient's transmitter is in a pouch with the microphone attached to a strap and the antenna threaded up into the strap. Wherever they first come together, the doctor merely drops the strap over the patient's head (who has previously signed a consent) so that the pouch is about midchest height. This is not an inexpensive or trouble-free method. The recording quality must be checked at least daily. Batteries must constantly be checked, and antennae tend to cause difficulties. However, vigilance is rewarded with broadcast quality recording. Recorders can be stopped and started from the Sennheiser transmitter, but this is chancy because often the physician forgets to restart the tape recorder when appropriate. Where possible, it is better to have a member of the doctor's staff or the recording team control the machine. This is sophisticated equipment which, while demanding, is not difficult to use if one is patient and follows the instructions carefully. For recording lesser volumes of conversation, a stereophonic cassette machine with two microphones on long cords will be sufficient.

Do not worry that the microphones will intimidate the patients. They have come to the doctor with a purpose, and the microphone is usually seen as a small inconvenience. On occasion, however, a patient may hold back because of the recording. You should always be alert to this possibility so that if you become aware of his or her hesitation, you can offer to stop the recording. Do not be too quick to do that, however, it is the patient's hesitancy not yours that is important. On occasion a patient will take advantage of the microphone to deliver a sermon about medical care. That seems only fair. One patient, left stranded on an examining table with the transmitter around his neck, used the opportunity to complain humorously, but pointedly, about the trials of waiting and the importance of time to patients as well as doctors. Doctors, on the other hand, often require considerable reassurance before they will wear microphones. They seem convinced that everyone is waiting to catch them in some gaffe or to demonstrate how badly they communicate. I believe that teaching by negative example is not as effective as demonstrating the principles of good communication. Therefore, with some exceptions, I am not particularly interested in showing my colleagues what they, in particular, are doing "wrong." They might find it rewarding if you give them copies of their own tapes.

Buy the best tape that your budget will allow. Fortunately excellent tape that will suffice for voice recording is considerably less expensive than that required for music. It is frequently possible to purchase non-brand-name cassettes or reel-to-reel tape from reliable wholesalers which is considerably less expensive and of equal quality. Cassettes that play longer than ninety minutes have more troubles than shorter cassettes and should be avoided. The cassette cartridge should be the type that can be dissembled in case of difficulty.

Keep the equipment clean and well maintained. Microphones should be treated like delicate instruments—expensive to purchase and costly to repair. Demagnetize the recorder heads frequently. Properly cleaned and aligned tape recorders play and record significantly better, but real skill is required for these tasks. When large volumes of recordings are to be made, find a reliable technician for the maintenance tasks.

I have not found it useful to transcribe recordings routinely into the written word. There are several reasons for this. First, it requires about eight hours of typing time for each hour of recorded conversation. Second, accurate transcription is a demanding task if the transcriber is to avoid errors. Third, no single method of transcription exists that accurately represents speech on the printed page and can be easily read. Several transcription systems have been devised, but they are so time-consuming and demand so much expertise to write and to read that they are not practical except for very small amounts of recording or special purposes. Most important, however, is the fact that the spoken language is different from written language, and it should be studied in its original form. Any time that transcribed speech becomes the object of research rather than the original recording, the investigator must be aware that a potentially misleading artifact has been introduced. The reason often given for transcribing —maintaining access to the material—is easily accomplished by good cataloging methods.

Because it has become such a simple matter to record the interactions between doctors and patients, one readily accumulates tapes. Unfortunately six hours of recordings require six hours of listening, sixty hours require sixty hours, and ad infinitum. (There are cassette players that permit accelerating the tape speed while maintaining pitch. One can learn to listen with these at rates almost double real time, though it requires practice.) Only an adequate cataloging system will prevent drowning in tape. The most commonly employed method, the doctor's memory, is totally inadequate for more than ten or so hours of recordings (and even then only if the tape has been listened to many times). Retrieval of recorded information may not seem important when a tape is being made, but searching for a specific piece of data months later on inadequately cataloged tapes can be maddening. The key to the success of the project on which this book is based was the ability to know the content of the recordings. The methods described are quite general in nature and with some modification should meet most needs.

Aside from the most general categories, catalog entries are most accurate and easily retrived when they refer to time elapsed from the beginning of a tape. Tape-recorder revolution counters are often used to demarcate catalogs, but because they refer to nothing "real" like time or tape length, numbers on the revolution counter of the tape recorder can only be used as a tempory substitute for elapsed time. Calibration will be different for each type of recorder and may even differ for machines of the same make and model. Accurate calibration to one minute is sufficient for rough purposes, but a minute is a long time to listen through while searching for a specific place on the tape;

therefore calibration to ten-second accuracy will repay the initial investment in working time.

For example, when a set of office hours is being recorded, a log should be made that will permit entering the patient's name, the time the interaction started, and the time it ended, with space for comments about what transpired during the visit. In place of, or in addition to, the comments it may be useful to list subjects discussed during the visit in terms of your own interests. Our logs might contain words such as, "pain," "heart disease," "weight loss," "grief," indicating that such topics came up during a visit. These entries should be made while the recording is in progress, rather than afterwards when things are quickly forgotten. Similar entries can be done for cassette recording. Thus a minimal catalog will contain (1) an identifying number for the reel of tape or the cassette, (2) the name of each patient, and (2a) doctor, if different doctors are recorded on a single tape, (3) the time the interaction with each patient started and ended, measured from the beginning of the cassette or reel, (4) subject matter considered worthy of noting, each item identified by one word or brief phrase, contained in the interaction. Such a catalog should be made while recording is in progress.

A more complete catalog can be constructed while listening to a tape, and often (after some experience) at normal listening speed. The same principles are followed. The far left column of the cataloging page (see figure 1) provides space for entering the elapsed time from the beginning of the tape to all other entries in the catalog. The next column is for the speaker. An entry should be made every time the speaker changes. Another column is reserved for the content of the participant's conversation entered as single words or brief phrases. One column may be employed to record specific affects such as laughing or crying.

Each person or group that records doctor-patient interactions has some special interest that will be reflected in their choice of material to be cataloged. As you can see from the sample catalog page from our research, we were initially interested in a modified speech-act theory. Thus our catalogs recorded the speech acts of the participants. Such special interests generally reflect a theoretical approach to the study of, say, conversation or doctoring. They may be derived from the hypotheses on which the study is based. It is not unusual for such special interests, hypotheses, or ways of notating tape recording to fall from favor as time passes. If cataloging has been done entirely in these terms, the catalogs and the tapes themselves may entirely lose their future value. This is a pity because the tape recordings, if they are of

ADDRESS	SPKR	MAIN CONVERS DIV	SPEECH ACT	LEXICAL CONTENT	MISC	ATTIT/AFFECT	CONVERSATIONAL CONTENT
0858	B		Suggesting Informing	WEAK BECAUSE LOST WEIGHT	SHARED INFORMATION		CAUSALITY, WEIGHT
0858	A	BANTER		NOT SO BAD			
0863	A			HOSPITAL EXPERIENCE			HOSPITALIZATION
0863	B			PLEASANT AS IT COULD BE			
0870					PHONE DIAL		APPOINTMENT, PAIN FEAR ABOUT BREAST
0903					CALLS END		
0906	A	INTERROG		WHAT DO YOU FEEL NOW			
				COMPARED to WEEK BEFORE	SHARED INFORMATION		
				WENT INTO HOSPITAL			
0909	B		HEDGING	EAT LATE			CAUSALITY
0910	A		GREETING	DON'T GIVE REASON, ASK			FEELINGS
				WHAT FEEL LIKE			
0913	B	NARRATIVE		WEAK - DON'T HAVE SHORTNESS OF BREATH - TRYING NOT to go up + down STAIRS			WEAKNESS
				APPETITE - diarrhea			SHORTNESS OF BREATH MEDICATION

Figure 1

natually occuring doctor-patient interactions, preserve something of enduring value that can often be restudied again and again with profit. Hence, whatever your special interests may be, you will be repaid if at least one or two columns of your catalog contain everyday language references to content. Videotape recordings can be cataloged in the same manner with added columns for visual material. These cataloging methods are unavoidably subjective—they cannot be otherwise. If different individuals are doing the cataloging, uniformity can only be approached by rigorous training, a thorough written manual, continuous supervision, constant quality checks, and frequent refresher training. On one occasion I reviewed a project in which two inexperienced investigators were rating physicians on a particular behavior based on videotapes of their consultations. They had developed criteria for cataloging the behavior exhibited on the videotapes which were to be followed by two catalogers hired for the purpose. The researchers had spent no time watching their own tapes or sitting in on doctors' consultations. They had fallen prey to the common error of establishing criteria in advance, often based on the findings or theory of others, for some phenomenon that is to be cataloged from the recordings without making sure that such criteria are true to the naturally occurring interactions or that they can be clearly identified while listening. There is no substitute for listening to many hours of recorded conversation before deciding what special phenomena should be cataloged. If you follow these methods, you will find that it is possible to maintain reasonably rapid access to specific items even in large volumes of recordings. These methods are also easily adapted to modern personal computer data-base programs so that you can automate storage and retrieval and not be at the mercy of institutional computer departments. I wish such equipment and software had been available when this project was in progress.

High quality tape recordings are a teaching resource of enormous value. Listening to a naturally occurring interaction, in which a doctor asks a patient a set of questions, teaches more about questioning than making the same point in a lecture. This is a variant of "one picture is worth a thousand words." For tape recordings to achieve their potential impact, however, they require editing. Long pauses, extraneous sounds, tangential digressions, embedded clauses, and redundacies are a part of natural conversation which usually do not bother participants. The same conversation quickly loses the attention of an audience. Thus, in order for a recorded example to maintain the engagement of a group of listeners at the same time that it makes a point, everything extraneous to that point should be edited out. One must be careful, however, not to edit in such a manner that the example no longer sounds like conversation or does not fairly represent the speakers. The last point is important. One must be fair to the patients and doctors who consent to be recorded and not distort their meanings or make them sound silly or foolish. There are no other hard and fast rules about editing because it is an aesthetic process. One wants the finished example to make its point parsimoniously and in a manner that maintains the interest of an audience. There are times when no shortcuts can be taken; the audience must listen to a long example in order to reach understanding. Be sparing of such occasions—what fascinates you may tire others—boredom rarely encourages learning.

Good editing requires good equipment. A reel-to-reel tape recorder with easy access to the playback head permits the editor to know with precision where on the tape a sound is to be found. By carefully marking the tape with pencils sold for the purpose and splicing accurately, sounds occupying fractions of a second can be removed or inserted. Many manipulations are possible that can enhance the teaching value of recordings. Sometimes examples can be simulated by having people act the parts and dubbing in appropriate background. The possibilities are limited only by imagination. One knows one has been successful when the completed examples sound just like natural conversation! Three other things are necessary: carefulness, patience, and time—especially time. An hour of finished taped examples may require forty hours or more to edit. I know of no shortcuts, but the end result can have such great teaching impact that the product is worth the effort. Cassettes cannot be edited in the same manner as reel-to-reel tape. Dubbing in sections from one cassette to another does not have the capacity for the same quality as splicing tape. Editing should be done on copies with the original recordings carefully protected. However, since each successive generation of copies loses fidelity, some noise reduction system such as Dolby or DBX is essential. It is very helpful in the beginning to have a knowledgeable editor demonstrate how things are done—and better yet to have an experienced person do the editing.

At whatever level of interest, from the desire to improve your communication with patients to the detailed study of the spoken language, high quality recordings that are carefully cataloged and that have been obtained with well maintained good equipment are a resource of lasting value.

Suggested Readings

Abercrombie, David. *Elements of General Phonetics*. Edinburgh: Edinburgh University Press, 1967.

Austin, J. L. *How To Do Things With Words*. New York: Oxford University Press, 1973.

Austin, J. L. *Philosophical Papers*. New York: Oxford University Press, 1970.

Bakan, David. *Pain, Disease and Sacrifice*. Chicago: University of Chicago Press, 1968.

Balint, M. *The Doctor, His Patient and the Illness*. 2nd Ed. London: Pitman Medical, 1964.

Bauman, R., and Sheizer, J., eds. *Explorations in the Ethnography of Speaking*. New York: Cambridge University Press, 1974.

Brown, Gillian. *Listening to Spoken English*. London: Longman, 1977.

Bruner, J. S. *Beyond the Information Given*. New York: W. W. Norton, 1973.

Byrne, P. S., and Long, B. E. L. *Doctors Talking to Patients*. London: Her Majesty's Stationary Office, 1976.

Cassell, Eric J. *The Healer's Art*. New York: Lippincott, 1976. Penguin, 1979.

Cassell, Eric J. *The Place of the Humanities in Medicine*. Hastings-on-Hudson: The Hastings Center, 1984.

Deutsch, F., and Murphy, W. F. *The Clinical Interview*. New York: International University Press, 1960.

De Villiers, J., and De Villiers, P. *Language Acquisition*. Cambridge, Mass.: Harvard University Press, 1978.

Enelow, A. J., and Swisher, Scott N. *Interviewing and Patient Care*. New York: Oxford University Press, 1972.

Fodor, J. A., Bever, T. G., and Garrett, M. F. *The Psychology of Language*. New York: McGraw-Hill, 1974.

Gordon, George N. *The Languages of Communication*. New York: Hastings House, 1969.

Halliday, M. A. K., and Hasan, R. *Cohesion in English*. London: Longman, 1975.

Halliday, M. A. K. *Language as Social Semiotic*. London: Arnold (Publishers), 1978.

Hardy, W. G. *Language, Thought and Experience*. Baltimore: University Park Press, 1978.

Hare, R. M. *The Languages of Morals*. New York: Oxford University Press, 1969.

Hayden, D. E., Alworth, E. P., and Tate, G. *Classics in Linguistics*. New York: Philosophical Library, 1967.

Hymes, Dell. *Foundations in Sociolinguistics*. Philadelphia: University of Pennsylvania Press, 1974.

Howell, R. W., and Vetter, H. J. *Language and Behavior*. New York: Human Sciences Press, 1976.

Jakobovits, L. A., and Miron, M. S., eds. *Readings in the Psychology of Language*. Englewood Cliff, N. J.: Prentice-Hall, 1967.

Judge, R. D., Zuidema, G. D., and Fitzgerald, F. T. *Clinical Diagnosis*. 4th Ed. Boston: Little Brown, 1982.

Labov, William. *Language in the Inner City*. Philadelphia: University of Pennsylvania Press, 1972.

Labov, William. *Sociolinguistic Patterns*. Philadelphia: University of Pennsylvania Press, 1972.

Labov, William, and Fanshel, David. *Therapeutic Discourse*. New York: Academic Press, 1977.

Ladefoged, Peter. *A Course in Phonetics*. New York: Harcourt Brace Jovanovich, 1975.

Lain-Entralgo, Pedro. *Doctor and Patient*. New York: McGraw-Hill (World University Library), 1969.

Lain-Entralgo, Pedro. *The Therapy of the Word in Classical Antiquity*. New Haven: Yale University Press, 1970.

Laver, John, and Hutcheson, Sandra, eds. *Communication in Face to Face Interaction*. Baltimore: Penguin, 1972.

Lyons, John, ed. *New Horizons in Linguistics*. Baltimore: Penguin, 1970.

Lyons, John. *Introduction to Theoretical Linguistics*. Cambridge: Cambridge University Press, 1968.

Lyons, John. *Semantics*. Vols. 1 and 2. Cambridge: Cambridge University Press, 1977.

Lyons, John. *Language Meaning and Context*. London: Fontana, 1981.

McIntosh, J. *Communication and Awareness on a Cancer Ward*. New York: Prodist, 1977.

Miller, George A. *Language and Communication*. New York: McGraw-Hill, 1951.

Miller, George A., and Johnson-Laird, Philip N. *Language and Perception*. Cambridge, Mass. Belknap Press, 1976.

Ozer, Mark N. *Solving Learning and Behavior Problems of Children*. San Francisco: Jossey-Bass, 1980.

Percy, Walker. *The Message in the Bottle*. New York: Farrar, Straus and Giroux, 1978.

Richardson, S. A. Dohrenwend, B. S. and Klein, D. *Interviewing*. New York: Basic Books, 1965.

Rochester, Sherry, and Martin, J. R. *Crazy Talk: A Study of the Discourse of Schizophrenic Speakers*. New York: Plenum, 1979.

Schiffer, S. R. *Meaning*. Oxford: Clarendon, 1974.

Searle, J. R. *Speech Acts*. Cambridge: Cambridge University Press, 1969.

Watzlawick, Paul. *How Real is Real*. New York: Vintage Books, 1976.

Watzlawick, P., and Beavin, J. H., and Jackson, D. D. *Pragmatics of Human Communication*. New York: W. W. Norton, 1967.

Index